# What Can During Intermittent Fasting?

# The Science of Fasting Explained

Mag. Stephan Lederer, Bakk., MSc

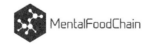

www.mentalfoodchain.com

This book is designed as an informational resource only. The information contained in this book should in no way be considered a substitute for the advice of a qualified physician, who should always be consulted before beginning any new diet, workout, or other health programs. Every effort has been made to ensure the accuracy of the information contained in this book at the time of publication. The author expressly disclaims responsibility for any adverse effects resulting from the use or application of the information contained in this book.

*This book is dedicated to those people who
like to pour themselves pure coffee
and develop their personality
a small step every day.*

# Contents

# Introduction

Fasting is simple. It means not feeding the body with food.

At first glance, this principle sounds simple, but appearances are deceptive. Behind the supposedly simple nutritional concept are complex processes that the human body goes through.

Our everyday actions influence those processes that make up intermittent fasting, often without us noticing.

Only one thing can help against unconscious mistakes that destroy the health progress of intermittent fasting: a solid basic understanding of how food intake affects metabolism during fasting.

I have learned from hundreds of thousands of readers that the drinks during fasting raise countless questions.

If someone begins with the allegedly simple diet, questions arise, which so far still nobody could answer completely:

- What am I allowed to drink during intermittent fasting?
- Is coffee with milk allowed?
- Can I drink tea with sweetener?
- Is lemon water allowed?
- What about diet soda?

Have you already asked yourself similar questions? If so, you've come to the right place.

This book has set out to clarify once and for all what drinks are allowed during Intermittent Fasting.

Since the topic is neither quickly settled nor old news, we'll be basing this on recent studies.

But don't worry. My main goal is to give you the information in clear, simple terms that will make it easy to use in your everyday life.

# Intermittent Fasting 101

Intermittent fasting involves eating within a certain period and fasting the rest of the day.

Although there are various forms of intermittent fasting, the most popular form of fasting is abstaining from food for a 16-hour window.

On the other hand, drinking is allowed around the clock and essential, as more water leaves your body than before, especially in the beginning.

What you can drink during intermittent fasting without breaking the fast and negating the health benefits will be explained in detail in the course of this book.

# Plans and Methods

Intermittent fasting methods are as individual as the people who use them.

That is why there is a wide variety of intermittent fasting protocols, which can have significant differences. Accordingly, different plans also have individual advantages and disadvantages.

Let's find out together what characteristics the different methods have and their advantages and disadvantages to your individual everyday life.

## Intermittent Fasting 16/8

Although various forms of intermittent fasting exist, the most popular is eating within a window of about 8 hours. We will take a closer look at why this is so soon.

The classic 16/8 method is also known as *time-restricted eating, peak fasting, or lean-gains method* because it allows you to gain muscle mass while losing body fat.

Therefore, the standard intermittent fasting method is not a foreign word even in circles of bodybuilders since they have already been using it for decades.

For example, you eat thereby between noon and 8 PM. Therefore, the body can fast for 16 hours with an 8-hour eating period in between. Since you sleep 8 out of the 16 fasting hours, classic Intermittent fasting is more convenient than you might think.

You can also successfully use this method with a 14, 18, or 20-hour fasting window or approach more extended periods depending on your daily routine.

However, the classic fasting interval remains 16/8:

- **Fasting window:** 16 hours
- **Feeding window:** 8 hours

## One Meal A Day (OMAD)

The OMAD Diet is not a diet but rather a more extreme form of the 16/8 intermittent fasting protocol.

Therefore, *One Meal A Day* means that you eat only once and fast the rest of the day. With this in mind, OMAD is not the proper method for beginners.

Therefore, for me, OMAD is more of a situational method for people who have been fasting with the 16/8 plan for a more extended time than a strict diet.

In my opinion, we just covered the most significant advantage of fasting. It's tremendously flexible. If you are busy and just in the workflow, you can skip lunch, save time, and 16/8 becomes OMAD without any additional effort.

Accordingly, OMAD is similar to 16/8. Hence, it is also called the 23/1 fasting method or 23/1 diet.

With the following fasting period, OMAD is even simpler than intermittent fasting 16/8:

- **Fasting window:** 23 hours
- **Feeding window:** 1 hour

## Alternate Day Fasting (ADF)

This method is just as simple as it sounds: eat one day, fast the other day.

However, most people eat a small meal (about 500 calories) on a fasting day. Therefore, although it is relatively widespread, this method is not a favorite of mine.

Not only does a small meal make you hungry, but it also negates the benefits of autophagy. We will learn more about why this process is so essential to the health benefits of fasting soon.

ADF is also more difficult to incorporate into daily routines than other methods.

In addition, many people abuse ADF because they think it allows them to maintain their *Standard American Diet (SAD)*, dominated by refined carbohydrates and sugar.

Therefore, ADF is usually unsuccessful since what you eat does matter, even with intermittent fasting. Moreover, low-quality diets can cause side effects such as headaches.

Nevertheless, this method is also surprisingly simple:

- **Fasting window:** 24 hours (incl. small meal)
- **Feeding window:** 24 hours

## 24-Hour-Fasting or 6:1 Diet

The better variant of alternate-day fasting is 24-hour fasting, also known as *eat-stop-eat* or *6:1 diet*. Here you strictly do not eat at all on one day per week.

Since you usually fast for two nights, the fasting period often lasts longer than 24 hours. From dinner to breakfast the day after next, it is usually 36 hours.

You can benefit more from the anti-aging effect of autophagy and burn body fat much more efficiently for energy.

Especially for athletes and people who don't want to restrict themselves daily, 1-day fasting is a popular option on a rest day:

- **Fasting window:** 24 to 40 hours
- **Feeding window:** Rest of the week

## 48-Hour-Fasting or 5:2 Diet

In the standard version of the 5:2 diet, calorie intake is limited to 500 calories per day for two consecutive days per week (with two meals of 250 calories each).

The remaining five days of the week, you eat regularly. For example, you could eat only 500 calories per day on Monday and Tuesday and normally eat Wednesday through Sunday.

Although eating small meals may seem easier at first to approach fasting, it destroys the results.

When insulin levels rise, the hormone inhibits fat burning, autophagy, and related beneficial effects.

In addition, small meals will not satiate at all and instead initiate cravings.

Since the hunger hormone ghrelin decreases with fasting, it is wiser to fast without a snack.[1]

In my opinion, it is, therefore, a better alternative to go on a strict 24-hour fast. This approach gives the digestive tract a well-deserved break, cleanses the body, and makes it easier for you to burn fat.

Furthermore, it is far more practical to limit fasting to one day of the week. If you can fit two nights into the fasting period, that's, of course, even better. After all, fasting is incredibly comfortable while you sleep.

Moreover, it is even more efficient for cell renewal to fast strictly for 48 hours. Nevertheless, this duration is not suitable for starting.

Furthermore, fasting periods of 48+ hours are better used selectively as therapeutic fasting methods than to put the body under additional stress regularly. The schedule of the 5:2 diet is composed as follows:

- **Fasting window:** 48 hours (incl. small meals)
- **Feeding window:** 5 days of the week

# Why 16 Hours of Fasting?

Now that we have learned about the colorful variety of intermittent fasting, you may wonder why a fasting period over 16 hours has become popular.

Shouldn't weight loss increase in effectiveness with the duration of fasting?

With this in mind, indeed, more extreme methods such as OMAD or strict 5:2 fasting might be more powerful. The reason for the popularity of the 16/8 schedule is the balance of two essential factors in fasting:

- Activation of autophagy
- Integration into everyday life

On the one hand, there are practical reasons for the 16 hours of intermittent fasting. Once you skip breakfast or even dinner, you extend the natural fasting period. Hence, you can reach a fasting period of 16 hours without much effort.

For a good reason, you might have heard that people lose weight mainly while sleeping because this is the last fasting period we have left today, thanks to conventional diet advice.

Eating from noon to 8 PM is enormously comfortable because the hunger in the morning is just learned. You will notice this fact two weeks after you start 16/8 at the latest.

In addition, our body injects us with a cocktail of hormones in the morning that provides sufficient energy for the day ahead. Because primarily cortisol, adrenaline, and growth hormones reach peak levels in the morning, we wake up.

Besides, skipping breakfast allows us always to have dinner with our loved ones. Since dinner is an essential social cornerstone of many families, this method conveniently fits into most daily routines.

Nevertheless, it doesn't mean that you have to skip breakfast. You can also do the 16/8 method by skipping dinner. Finally, intermittent fasting is flexible, and you can adapt it to your unique routine.

Unlike these two variants, skipping lunch is less effective.

Why is that?

Therefore, we have to tackle autophagy, the second essential factor for the 16 hours.

Since this recycling process in human cells is responsible for many remarkable health benefits of fasting, its discovery was even honored with the Nobel Prize in Medicine.[2]

According to recent studies, people need an average of about 14 hours without meals to activate autophagy in their bodies significantly.[3]

Thus, we have found the second essential argument for 16 hours in intermittent fasting. Accordingly, the 16/8 protocol is the perfect trade-off of comfort and health benefits that has been established over the years.

Although about two hours of proper cellular cleansing may seem manageable right off the bat, we must remember that the anti-aging effect is repeated daily and eventually adds up.

However, you can speed up the process by exercising, eating a low-carb or, even better, a ketogenic diet, increasing autophagy effectiveness during the 16 hours.

I will explain in more detail why autophagy is so crucial in the second section of this book.

But first, we will address significant mistakes by which intermittent fasting beginners repeatedly prevent results or cause unpleasant side effects.

# Top 5 Intermittent Fasting Mistakes

At the beginning of a new routine, every person goes through a learning process. The process includes making mistakes because only from these can be learned.

Nevertheless, I want to save you time at this point and explain five common mistakes that intermittent fasting beginners usually make entirely unconsciously.

The exciting thing is that except for one of these common mistakes, all of them have to do with drinking. For this reason, the question about the allowed drinks is so essential when it comes to fasting.

## 1. Too Little Activity

A persistent myth about fasting is that you must always take it easy, especially if you feel tired.

If you already feel tired, the surest way to eventually feel terrible is to rest even more. Instead, activity can help the body go to fat-burning more efficiently.

After our bodies try to conserve energy where they can, fat-burning often requires physical activity to get it going.

If you feel fatigued while fasting, it's often a sign that carbohydrate stores are depleting. However, we can't burn fat until these short-term batteries are empty.

Then the human body tells us with sluggishness that quickly available energy is running low. However, it does not want to expend additional metabolic energy for burning body fat right away.

Accordingly, body fat is like a savings account only tackled when the checkings account (our carbohydrate stores in the liver and skeletal muscles) is empty.[4]

That's why it helps to increase your energy needs with exercise. This way, you force your body to switch to burning body fat.

Another mistake is to overdo it with an intense workout. On the other hand, a leisurely walk or even yoga will help to boost fat burning.

Nonetheless, it is crucial to listen to your body when fasting. If you feel good with fasting and more intensive weight lifting, go for it.

However, since fasting doesn't run away from you, you can always break your fast when you feel uncomfortable doing it.

For me, strength training and intermittent fasting work very well. This is partly because, during fasting, an exceptionally high amount of growth hormone is released, which otherwise could not be achieved.

Accordingly, the proper coordination of intermittent fasting and resistance training promotes muscle growth.

It is different regarding intensive endurance training, such as marathon preparation. In my experience, the body's increased appetite and need for recovery speak against more extended periods of fasting.

As long as you feel sluggish, however, the following tips can help you:

- **Exercise:** If you feel low on energy, don't stop moving altogether. Otherwise, you'll become even more sluggish. So grab the bike or take the dog for a walk.

- **Activity:** Treat the fasting day or period like any other. Although fasting beginners are usually nervous, it's no big deal. Nature designed our bodies for it. Housework or gardening can distract you and keep you active.

- **Measure:** If you have a fatigue attack, a 15-minute walk can help.

## 2. Too Little Salt

Apart from fat, hardly anything has been demonized as much as salt for decades. Not only advertising campaigns but also doctors have caused this distorted image. Nevertheless, salt is not as bad as its reputation.

Few people are aware that we cannot survive without salt. Although a daily requirement of two grams is currently recommended, our ancestors instinctively consumed 2-3 times as much salt.

Amazingly, even today, the countries with the highest salt consumption have the lowest rates of cardiovascular disease.[5]

In addition, salt is the natural antagonist of sugar, takes the bitter taste out of our food, and works against cravings.

Unlike sugar, salt has a negative feedback loop. When your body has had enough salt, you don't crave it anymore.

For example, I have trouble eating salty soup. With cake and sugar, however, things are different. Sound familiar?

Moreover, recent studies suggest that too little salt intake may be more harmful to our health than the other way around.

Accordingly, endocrinologist and fasting pioneer, Dr. Jason Fung, reports that physical side effects of fasting are usually due to too little salt consumption.

For example, he says, these are especially headaches and dizziness.

Furthermore, he has observed in his diabetes clinic that salt intake is essential for weight loss, especially in women. In this context, we must also note that salt can help prevent type 2 diabetes.[6]

While sugar consumption promotes insulin resistance and body fat storage, salt increases insulin sensitivity and helps you lose weight instead.[7]

Good options for getting healthy salt into your diet include pink Himalayan salt or Celtic sea salt. Since these salts usually don't contain chemical additives like anti-caking agents, they are more natural.

Nevertheless, as with any other dietary change, it is

essential to consult with your trusted physician.

In cases of chronic kidney disease or certain cardiovascular diseases, people need to watch their sodium intake.

If you experience headaches while fasting, the following home remedies can help:

- **Salt to taste:** Listen to your body and dare to salt food properly when it asks for it.

- **Drink bone broth:** Many fasting beginners find it helpful to drink bone broth or unsweetened pickle juice until the body gets used to the lifestyle.

- **Use sole water:** If you don't have sugar-free pickle juice or bone broth on hand, dissolve a pinch of salt in a glass of water — the same works with tea or coffee.

- **Cut back on carbohydrates:** Carbohydrates retain water in the body. If you eat bread, cookies, protein, or granola bars between fasts, water will be stored and then flushed out along with sodium, causing headaches.

## 3. Poor Diet

Although beginners are often afraid of not getting enough nutrients during intermittent fasting, in my experience, this is somewhat unjustified.

During fasting, the hormone system sets the course

for fat burning. However, this does not mean you have to eat less. Instead, you get your nutrients more concentrated in two larger meals.

Nevertheless, you are still responsible for the quality of the food you eat.

If you have just started intermittent fasting, your body flushes excess water and electrolytes out through the gastrointestinal tract.

But that is nothing to worry about and can also have several other triggers such as excessive caffeine consumption from tea or coffee.

Hence, you have to ensure essential electrolytes such as potassium, magnesium, and sodium through your diet.

Nonetheless, intermittent fasting will not cause diarrhea in the long run.

Instead, you are likely to get diarrhea if you break the fast. But that is a natural reaction when the gastrointestinal tract starts working again after an extended fasting period.

However, if this condition persists for an extended time with a consistent fasting window, it's much more likely that you're simply eating poorly.

Many people's intestines struggle with the following usual suspects:

- Refined carbohydrates
- Legumes high in fiber and lectins
- Too much dairy (lactose and beta-casein A1)

Those who base their fasting diet on baking goods, sweets, beans, and low-fat dairy products could cause noticeable complications. In addition, you will hardly lose weight with such a diet.

In addition to one extreme of diarrhea, the other extreme of constipation can occur due to a diet affluent in fiber.

Since fiber is that part of plant food that the body cannot digest, it increases stool volume.

And as researchers have now correctly recognized, it isn't easy to pass large volumes through a narrow opening.

Nonetheless, some people still believe they can prevent constipation by increasing fiber intake.

But studies show that the exact opposite is true.[8]

In addition to reducing the above foods, the following beverages can help you with digestive problems:

- **Water:** Increased water consumption is always welcome and necessary to prevent dehydration.

- **Bone broth:** When suffering from diarrhea, increased electrolyte intake through drinks such as bone broth, pickle juice, or sole water is essential.

- **Other drinks:** Avoid sugary, caffeinated, and diet soda.

## 4. Too Little Water

A common mistake in intermittent fasting is that people like to confuse thirst with hunger.

Instead of reaching for water or tea, we go for a protein bar since solid food also provides fluid to a certain degree.

When we forgo familiar snacks, however, we often don't replenish the fluids they gave us.

As a result, we think we feel hungry. Accordingly, during periods of fasting and between meals, you often don't crave food but simply a craving for fluid that needs to be satisfied.

Accordingly, some people need regular reminders in their daily lives to take in enough fluids.

So how much do you need to drink during a fasting period?

Fluid intake during intermittent fasting cannot be generalized.

Neither do utopian recommendations of 5 liters of water per day apply to everyone, nor can you calculate fluid needs based on weight, height, and age.

Moreover, overhydration is just as harmful as dehydration. Nevertheless, a simple rule of thumb applies: drink when you are thirsty.

As is often the case, it is better to listen to your body. If you're not thirsty, you don't have to force yourself to drink all the time. The same should apply to everyday life.

When in doubt, a glass of water or tea won't hurt. With more extended periods of fasting and experience, you will get a better sense of when you are thirsty.

The following options are available to counteract any hunger pangs you may feel in between meals:

- **Mineral water:** The carbonic acid in mineral water helps alleviate hunger pangs. Moreover, it replenishes electrolytes your body loses through urine.

- **A glass of water:** Drink a cup of tea or a glass of water when you feel hungry and wait 30 minutes. If hunger subsides, you are just thirsty.

- **Reminders:** If you have trouble drinking enough fluids, use your cell phone alarm clock for regular reminders.

## 5. Milk in Your Coffee

We have saved the most common mistake for last. Ultimately, this book deals with the effects of beverages on fasting because it is precisely there that most mistakes happen.

When drinking water, coffee, or tea, unintended mistakes repeatedly happen during intermittent fasting. But in most cases, people usually only lack reliable information.

Thus, many fasting beginners get carried away,

perhaps adding a splash of milk or a packet of sugar to their coffee.

But these subtle little things can have significant effects. By raising blood sugar and insulin levels, they break the fast. So, time and time again, a good portion of the health benefits and, more importantly, the progress in losing weight are negated.

For example, ketogenic diet followers tend to forget that a so-called *Bulletproof Coffee* also breaks the fast.

So butter, coconut, or MCT oil in the coffee helps against hunger in between but prevents the full health effect of fasting.

Although bone broth is a prime source of electrolytes and fat, it too technically breaks the fast and should only be used as a jump start. Once you get used to intermittent fasting, it is taboo or no longer necessary anyway, just like Bulletproof Coffee.

Moreover, many people don't know that while diet soda is sugar-free, that doesn't automatically mean it can't break a fast.

In addition, sweeteners stimulate cravings in the brain's reward center. So with the wide variety of options we have, it quickly becomes clear that the question of which beverages are allowed during intermittent fasting is not easy to answer.

The supposedly simple topic is highly complex. For this reason, I will explain to you what happens in the body during a fast, based on studies and yet in simple terms.

With this basic knowledge, we can then look at which drinks are allowed during intermittent fasting and the ones to avoid.

# How Do Beverages Affect Fasting?

To assess what you can drink during intermittent fasting, we must first elicit the reason for which we are fasting in the first place.

In short, there are two main reasons for intermittent fasting:

- Weight loss
- Autophagy

Although losing weight also causes health benefits, most of the positive effects of fasting in our bodies are supported by the process of autophagy.

With this in mind, we must emphasize that both fat burning and autophagy require low insulin levels.

## Weight Loss

There is a good reason why people can achieve outstanding weight loss results with intermittent fasting. Fasting is the most effective way to lower insulin levels.

Insulin is the essential storage hormone of the human body.

It is responsible for signaling cells to take up glucose from the bloodstream and store excess energy as fat or glycogen.

In addition, insulin blocks the enzyme that breaks down body fat.[9]

Accordingly, researchers can now predict about 75% of possible gains and losses in overweight people using insulin levels.[10]

The 16-hour fasting window cuts off the nutrient intake, lowers insulin levels, and thus ends the body's storage mode.

For this reason, the body can begin breaking down carbohydrates stored in the form of glycogen. Once glycogen stores are empty, your body can tap into stored fat for energy production.

This process of efficient fat burning is called ketosis and, contrary to popular myths, is an entirely natural mechanism that has ensured the survival of our species.

Nature has designed the body to build up fat reserves in times of abundance to draw from body fat in food shortages.

Now that we are experiencing an endless summer instead of food shortages and eat around the clock, we gain weight.

For this reason, intermittent fasting can help restore the natural balance between feeding and fasting, thereby normalizing insulin levels.

Ultimately, obesity is a hormonal imbalance rather than a caloric one, as the world-renowned neuroendocrinologist Dr. Robert Lustig concludes.[11]

# Autophagy

Autophagy is our body's mechanism for sorting out and recycling dysfunctional organelles, proteins, and cell membranes.

When there is not enough energy supply to sustain these decayed cellular parts, autophagy kicks in.

However, this is a regulated, orderly process of degradation and recycling of cellular components.

In this context, autophagy has three primary tasks in our cells:

- Remove defective proteins and organelles
- Remove pathogens
- Prevent atypical protein accumulation

Because he was able to demonstrate groundbreaking health benefits, the Japanese Yoshinori Ohsumi was awarded the Nobel Prize in Medicine for the discovery of this process.[12]

When food is scarce, the body goes from growth mode to maintenance mode. It then starts this intracellular recycling system, which breaks down broken cell parts and directs toxins out of the body.

But what does it depend on whether a drink inhibits or even ends autophagy?

To this end, three essential nutrient sensors exist in our bodies. Simply put, they switch the process of autophagy on and off:

- **Insulin:** Sensitive to carbohydrates and proteins.

- **mTOR:** Sensitive to proteins

- **AMPK:** Sensitive to lack of energy in cells

In this process, AMP-activated protein kinase (AMPK) responds when cells are supplied with energy, regardless of the macronutrient. Therefore, in addition to carbohydrates and proteins, fat also impairs autophagy.

Hence, both AMPK and insulin activate the mammalian target of rapamycin (mTOR).

Therefore, this enzyme, which is essential for growth, is called the primary nutrient sensor in our body. As soon as you eat, it detects nutrient availability and overrides autophagy.

However, if nutrient supply is interrupted for longer,

cells want to act sustainably and use defective cell parts for energy production.

If we now look at details on what to drink during intermittent fasting, autophagy is the benchmark.

Since the nutrient sensors governing autophagy also include insulin, it covers all the mechanisms that can break a fast.

Now that we have talked about the processes that initiate them in detail, it is time to learn about the main health benefits of fasting.

## Health Benefits

If you don't interrupt it unintentionally, interesting processes happen in the body during intermittent fasting, which has enriched the understanding of biochemistry and medicine with new insights over the past years.

Nevertheless, we have only touched on a fraction of the positive effects. Therefore, here are the ten most important health benefits that intermittent fasting sets in motion.

# 1. Anti-Aging

Every vehicle must be cared for and regularly maintained to function in excellent quality for as long as possible.

Therefore, fasting is the best way to keep your body in shape through autophagy.[13]

Once this intracellular recycling system is at work, it prevents the diseases that plague our Western society:

- Dementia, Alzheimer's and Parkinson's[14]
- Muscle and bone atrophy[15]
- Cardiovascular diseases[16]
- Insulin resistance and type 2 diabetes[17]
- Cancer[18]

In addition, research is increasingly unraveling that autophagy is also likely to renew damaged proteins and organelles in cardiac cells.[19]

Moreover, since it can slow down the aging process in general, autophagy is probably the most convincing reason to fast for at least 16 hours.[20]

# 2. Reduced Inflammation

Aging is defined as the accumulation of cellular damage with a decreasing ability to repair it. As a result, aging fundamentally causes some degree of inflammation in the body.

Recent studies suggest that fasting-induced autophagy can significantly slow this aging process and increase lifespan.[21]

Therefore, intermittent fasting also achieves remarkable results in the treatment of age-related diseases.

Moreover, intermittent fasting can reduce the need for proteins in the diet, as the body thereby recycles proteins from broken cell parts. This fact again has a positive effect on longevity.

Against this background, it is precisely widespread modern diseases such as arteriosclerosis, cancer, or type 2 diabetes characterized by too much growth and proteins.

In addition to autophagy, which breaks down defective proteins and protein accumulation, reducing inflammation in the body contributes to increased longevity.

Furthermore, ketosis during fasting lowers blood sugar and insulin levels, reducing inflammation and free radicals in the body that cause disease.

Therefore, another recent study notes the increase in life expectancy as a direct effect of intermittent fasting.[22]

## 3. Improved Cognition

In the brain, too, intermittent fasting can help break down accumulations of toxic proteins that promote dementia.

Accordingly, scientists found that in the early stages of dementia, the process of autophagy is significantly low.[23]

However, if ketones are burned from the fat stores instead of glucose from the carbohydrate stores through fasting or working out, signaling pathways increasing learning and memory function are activated.

Intermittent fasting can thus counteract neurodegenerative diseases such as Parkinson's or Alzheimer's disease.[24]

One of these signal generators is the neuronal growth hormone BDNF (brain-derived neurotrophic factor), which is responsible for forming new nerve cells.

Therefore, high BDNF levels are also associated with increased intelligence and memory function.

When you release BDNF, your brain can form new neural connections. For example, according to studies, fasting could improve memory in older people.[25]

In this context, the sympathetic nervous system is also activated, and the body releases adrenaline, cortisol, and growth hormones.

This fact could be another reason why many people

report increased cognition and awareness when fasting.

Hence, studies have not found a reduction in cognition in people who fasted for two days straight.[26]

Only breaking the fast allows the body to relax. Thus, the mental focus also fades again. You may have already noticed this circumstance as sluggishness after the meal.

# 4. Boosted Metabolism

Contrary to the myth that intermittent fasting slows down metabolism, scientists have long proven that it boosts it instead.[27]

Because fasting releases growth hormones and adrenaline, our ancestors were able to forage longer for food, precisely when it was scarce.

That's why they were able to ensure the survival of the species even during food shortages.[28]

Consequently, intermittent fasting increases the efficiency with which your body can tap into stored fat for energy.

In addition, the release of hormones such as norepinephrine keeps the basal metabolic rate up.[29]

## 5. Improved Muscle Gain

Intermittent fasting is no stranger to bodybuilding either. Classic time-restricted eating, in which you do not eat for 14 to 18 hours a day, is a proven method to gain lean mass.

Thereby, it is crucial to work out in a fasted state. Exercising on an empty stomach promotes not only autophagy but also fat burning.

Contrary to popular belief, muscles do not atrophy at all during fasting.

As we have already heard, intermittent fasting increases the release of growth hormones.

Thus, during fasting, not only muscle but also bone mass is protected from degeneration.[30]

Accordingly, targeted intermittent fasting in combination with appropriate training is an effective natural method for improved muscle gains.[31]

## 6. Enhanced Fat Burning

Intermittent fasting aims to burn fat as a primary source of energy during the fasting periods.

When released fatty acids from body fat or food enter the liver, they are converted into ketones to provide energy for the body. This metabolic process is therefore called ketosis.

Hence, fasting is the ultimate ketogenic diet because the body can only obtain energy from body fat without food intake.

For this reason, ketosis induced by intermittent fasting can burn fat reserves remarkably quickly.[32]

Furthermore, ketosis helps regulate appetite and stabilize blood sugar, which supports intermittent fasting and weight loss.

Accordingly, energy from ketones does not cause blood sugar to spike, as it does after high-carbohydrate meals. In addition, because ketones can cross the blood-brain barrier, they can provide sustained, clean mental energy.[33]

## 7. Less Visceral Fat

Intermittent fasting not only burns visually unflattering fat deposits.

Against this background, current studies state that intermittent fasting burns dangerous visceral fat more effectively than low-carb diets.[34]

Visceral fat deposits are fat accumulations in and around vital organs, such as the liver, intestines, or pancreas. There they lay the origin for secondary diseases.

Intra-organic fat contributes to non-alcoholic fatty liver disease, type 2 diabetes, and cardiovascular disease.[35]

Since the liver is the first place where malignant fat accumulates, it is often the root of modern metabolic diseases such as insulin resistance.

## 8. Improved Insulin Sensitivity

The scientific record of the effect of fasting against insulin resistance dates back to 1969.[36]

Also, today, studies refer to intermittent fasting as a safe treatment for insulin resistance.[37]

Insulin resistance is nothing more than a protective mechanism against the vast amounts of insulin caused by the *Wester Pattern Diet (WPD)* dominated by refined carbohydrates.

In this process, cells no longer respond appropriately to insulin, which prevents them from absorbing sufficient glucose from the bloodstream.

However, fat cells cannot become insulin resistant and blithely continue to store energy. Therefore, obesity is a significant symptom of the disease.

Besides combating the causative hyperinsulinemia, intermittent fasting can also reduce insulin resistance in the cells.

Thus, fasting can even reverse type 2 diabetes, the most significant secondary disease of insulin resistance, which diets alone usually cannot do.[38]

## 9. Increased Fertility

While excessive fasting may pose a threat for some women, properly executed intermittent fasting can positively affect fertility.

Polycystic ovarian syndrome (PCOS) is the most common metabolic disorder in women. It characterizes the development of cysts on the ovaries based on hormonal imbalance.

Like type 2 diabetes, obesity and hypertension are symptoms of PCOS. In short, it is even caused by severe insulin resistance, which also enormously increases the risk of diabetes in affected women.[39]

Nevertheless, in a recent study, intermittent fasting was able to help overweight women with PCOS. Because fasting increases the release of luteinizing hormone, it helps promote ovulation.

Furthermore, fasting, weight loss, and improved mental health may contribute to fertility.[40]

## 10. Improved Gut Health

Intermittent fasting is one of the best ways to improve gut health.

On the one hand, fasting periods allow the intestines to rest, and on the other hand, they starve out harmful gut bacteria.

But already, shorter fasting periods work. That's what a current study suggests, which determines an improved life expectancy due to short intermittent fasting periods at a young age.

In particular, reducing inflammation, which often has its origin in the gut, slows down the aging process.

Accordingly, intermittent fasting also reduces age-related diseases and strengthens the intestinal wall.[41]

Furthermore, intermittent fasting has the positive side effect of being able to improve food intolerances.

# What Am I Allowed to Drink During Fasting?

Humans can go without meals for over a year, but not without liquids. Accordingly, the world record for fasting under medical supervision is a whopping 382 days.[42]

Hydration is a particularly critical point in intermittent fasting. Ultimately, fasting aims to empty carbohydrate stores so that the body can burn stored fat for energy.

Since the body needs 3-4 grams of water per gram of carbohydrate to store it as glycogen in liver, kidney, and muscle cells, you will lose plenty of water during fasting.

Therefore, if you don't drink appropriately, you will experience the so-called keto flu symptoms, such as headaches or dizziness, during intermittent fasting.

These mild physical symptoms are primarily due to the lack of electrolytes, especially sodium, flushed out along with the water.

Therefore, although hydration is essential, you cannot provide it in all possible forms.

Why is this so?

Even the components of beverages can stimulate the three nutrient sensors in the body and stop autophagy and thus the health benefits of fasting.

Furthermore, if insulin is stimulated, the body can no longer draw on fat reserves for energy.

For this reason, we now examine a comprehensive selection of everyday drinks and deduce whether they can break a fast or not.

# Water

Fasting means not eating anything. Drinking water in its purest form, on the other hand, is not only permitted but also desired during interval fasting.

In addition to the necessary liquid, however, water can also provide the body with minerals naturally. In this case, however, the nutrient sensors are not activated, and do not break the fast.

Thus, tap water is, in any case, okay during intermittent fasting.

On the other hand, what about when the water comes from a mineral water source?

## Carbonated Water

When it comes to what you can drink during intermittent fasting, in my opinion, carbonated water is an outstanding choice.

On the one hand, it offers effects that excellently support intermittent fasting:

- It curbs the appetite,
- Helps with an upset stomach,
- Or even with cramping.

On the other hand, superior carbonated water can bring more than 100 mg per liter of the essential electrolytes, magnesium, sodium, and calcium, into your body.

Therefore, carbonated mineral water is the best choice. But only if you have access to natural, highly mineralized brands.

Here in Austria, we are blessed with incredible natural springs. But depending on where you are located, you might have to check labels carefully.

Hence, access to high-quality mineral water can provide electrolytes, even during extended fasts. In this case, you don't need to fall back to bone broth to get them.

## Flavored Sparkling Water

Although there is now flavored sparkling water with only natural flavorings, most products do not get by without sugar or sweeteners, which break the fast.

However, natural flavoring means that the flavoring agent has been extracted from a natural source by a chemical process.

Unless other additives are included, natural flavors can be limited to minimal macronutrients, so they hardly affect autophagy. Nevertheless, such products are still scarce.

In case of doubt, I would therefore not resort to flavored sparkling water. Besides, most flavored options taste artificial.

If you want to bring more flavor into your intermittent fasting plan, maybe natural flavors from fruits could get a variety in the water.

## Infused Water

If you want to flavor water, a natural way is probably generally better.

For example, you can put a few slices of organic

lime, lemon, orange, or cucumber in a carafe and fill it with water.

This way, you add a light natural aroma to the water that will not affect fasting significantly as long as you do not eat the slices.

However, this aid shouldn't be overused. Once you are used to intermittent fasting, you will be able to get along without it anyway.

## Lemon Water

In addition to the lemon slices, a small splash of lemon moves in a grey zone during intermittent fasting.

Suppose you want to be on the very safe side. In that case, it is better to leave a slice of organic lemon in the water, as the tiny amounts of calories come from carbohydrates, which technically can activate all three nutrient sensors.

Nonetheless, a splash of lemon will not negate all the benefits of fasting.

Since there is a low basic level of autophagy in the body at all times, it cannot be 100% deactivated immediately, especially not by relatively negligible amounts of macronutrients.

## Coconut Water

Many people believe in having found an excellent intermittent fasting drink in coconut water.

But that's not the case since the lion's energy share comes from sugar, unlike coconut.[43]

Furthermore, the proportion of electrolytes is much lower than one might think – no comparison to natural mineral water.

In summary, the supposedly natural coconut water fails as a drink during the fasting period.

Therefore, we can now focus on other beverages that share some characteristics with coconut water.

## Juices and Sodas

Advertising has been selling them as healthy since time immemorial.

Juices are often described as natural products and covered with organic, fair trade, and vegan labels.

But do juices, therefore, equal drinks that are suitable for a fasting cure?

## Juice

Compared to the consumption of whole foods, juices are way more harmful to health.

Since you remove the protective fiber with the flesh, juice leads to enormous blood sugar and insulin spikes.

Precisely because the dietary fibers' protective effect is missing, the fructose in fruit juices also bursts into the liver unchecked, causing insulin resistance and visceral fat in the long run.

For this reason, non-alcoholic fatty liver (NAFL) is much more common than fatty liver disease caused by alcohol.[44]

Fruit juice not only breaks the fast but is not much better than a coke – no matter how "organic" it is. Anyone who seriously wants to lose weight must keep their hands off it, even during eating periods.

## Celery Juice

Even though celery is on my low-carb food list, it remains a meal if you juice it.

Neither celery juice nor other vegetable juices are calorie-free, which breaks the fast. Moreover, it is precisely sugar that makes up the essential energy component in celery and stimulates insulin.[45]

## Smoothies

Although smoothies contain some fiber due to mixing instead of juicing, they break an intermittent fast.

Compared to fruit juices, they are the lesser evil but still represent a meal.

## Lemonade

Since it contains sugar, lemonade should not be drunk during intermittent fasting. Hence, you would have to reduce it to lemon water to be allowed during intermittent fasting.

We'll take a closer look at how the verdict looks regarding sugar-free sodas when we focus on sweeteners.

## Coffee

In my experience, coffee is the drink about which the most questions concerning intermittent fasting arise. Moreover, coffee is responsible for the most common mistakes during the fasting window.

However, this is no wonder. After all, coffee is a

faithful companion of many working people and a staple in many daily routines.

Although some religiously motivated fasting customs prohibit drinking coffee, it does not fundamentally harm intermittent fasting.

On the contrary, recent studies indicate that coffee does not inhibit autophagy but can even boost it.

Accordingly, scientists have found in mice that both caffeinated and decaffeinated coffee can activate autophagy in muscle tissue, liver, heart, and other major organs.[46]

Besides, according to a recent study, coffee drinkers can better maintain their weight in the long term.[47]

The fact that coffee reduces appetite could be a good reason for this.[48]

Moreover, since it increases the metabolic rate, coffee is particularly beneficial for weight loss.[49]

Therefore, the combination of coffee and intermittent fasting can help you last longer during your fast and lose weight faster.

Furthermore, drinking coffee while fasting can give your fat-burning an even more considerable boost because, according to recent research, coffee additionally enhances ketosis during fasting.[50]

In the long term, intermittent fasting is also an effective means of improving insulin sensitivity and thus glucose metabolism. For this reason, intermittent fasting helps prevent diabetes.

Nevertheless, fasting can decrease insulin sensitivity in the short term. On the other hand, since this reaction has a good reason, it is harmless.

In this way, the body ensures that most of the available glucose is supplied to the brain.

Therefore, other cells become acutely insulin resistant. So the brain parts that can't run on ketones and need glucose get enough of it.

However, you don't have to worry since the liver makes enough glucose from amino and fatty acids during fasting.[51]

Coffee has a similar effect. Acutely, coffee reduces insulin sensitivity and glucose tolerance. That is why the very combination of coffee and cake, which is part of good taste in our society, is poison when it comes to losing weight.

Nevertheless, coffee consumption improves insulin sensitivity and glucose metabolism in the long run. Thus, recent studies show that coffee consumption reduces the risk of type 2 diabetes.[52]

These numerous benefits underpin the importance of drinking coffee during intermittent fasting, which is why it will probably remain the most popular fasting drink, along with water and tea.

But how much coffee can you drink without breaking the fast?

## Black Coffee

One cup of black coffee may contain 1-4 calories and tiny amounts of protein, fat, and trace minerals.

Therefore, for most people, the nutrients in 1-2 cups of black coffee are not enough to affect the metabolism in a way that breaks the fast.[53]

Since coffee can help to suppress appetite, it also helps many people to last longer during fasting.

Due to the stimulation of the hormone adrenaline, which prepares our body for stressful situations, more significant amounts of coffee can influence intermittent fasting.[54]

This way, glucose may enter the bloodstream without food intake.[55]

As long as you do not drink more than 1-2 cups in a foreseeable timeframe, coffee will not inhibit autophagy in this indirect way.

Due to the following properties, you are allowed to have a cup of coffee now and then during fasting:

- It is rich in antioxidants that suppress appetite[56]
- Activates and supports autophagy[57]
- Increases metabolic rate[58]
- Supports sustainable weight loss[59]

Accordingly, espresso or plain coffee ideal for in-between meals when your appetite kicks in again. Still, it would help if you didn't consume lots of it.

Although there can be no generic answer here, I wouldn't drink more than 5 cups of coffee in a day.

And these should be spread throughout the day. That way, you're on the safe side. Rough amounts like 10 cups a day can affect fasting.

With 16/8 intermittent fasting, you can have 2-3 cups before lunch without any significant concerns.

But now comes the more exciting question. What additives are allowed in coffee during intermittent fasting?

## Coffee With Milk

100ml of milk not only contains almost 5g of lactose but also approximately as many milk proteins.

The calculation here is simple. With intermittent fasting, milk makes the difference in coffee. Even a dash of milk detracts from the benefits of fasting.

Coffee with milk breaks the fast. But what about skimmed milk?

## Skim Milk

Even with milk, the low-fat variant makes everything worse. As with other low-fat products, more sugar is hiding in skim milk. And, of course, there is less fat to counteract it.

In short, with skimmed milk, blood sugar and insulin levels rise even faster. That's why cereals with milk, for example, is one of the worst meals for your health – not only when you're on a ketogenic diet.

Also, skimmed milk is out. What about half and half?

## Half and Half

Since cream and regular milk can break a fast, half and half can too. Due to the significant mix of protein and carbs, half and half inhibits fasting benefits.

Furthermore, half and half is more likely to contain processed additives.

So regular kinds of milk are not safe for fasting. Can coffee with almond milk be an alternative for intermittent fasting?

## Cream

One hundred grams of heavy cream contain about three grams of milk sugar (lactose) and milk protein. Although some heavy cream does not necessarily inhibit fat burning, it will negatively affect autophagy.

Thus cream breaks a fast. However, that doesn't mean that a splash of cream destroys all the benefits. Fasting benefits such as autophagy do not have a binary switch. Nevertheless, heavy cream will inhibit results.

Nonetheless, heavy cream can be a welcome ingredient in a ketogenic diet since it helps to promote autophagy in the long run.

## Creamer

Creamer and similar additives in powder form are highly processed. Therefore, these are the ultimate junk foods!

They are loaded with carbohydrates, proteins, and fat. Moreover, some creamers consist of up to 50% sugar.

Also, coffee with sugar-free creamer isn't an option. Besides too much protein and fat, you will find other artificial additives like sweeteners in it.

If you like your body, you should avoid these junk additives not only during fasting.

## Almond Milk

Small amounts of unsweetened almond milk are in a grey zone during intermittent fasting. However, steer clear of soy- and rice-based almond drinks.

As long as you avoid the sweetened or protein-enriched versions and only add a shot, the effects of almond milk in coffee are negligible.

Nevertheless, almond milk technically breaks the

fast. Therefore pure nut milk is not suitable as a drink during fasting.

## Oat Milk

Since the food industry jumped on the vegan hype train, oat milk is currently enjoying great popularity.

But have you ever thought about the fact that it might be unnatural to make a milk substitute from grains? Where does the fat content come from, which you need for creaminess?

As I suspected, the fat in popular brands comes from industrially processed vegetable oils, such as canola oil.

To produce oil artificially from a non-oily plant is not only unnatural but also harms your health significantly.

Since chemical processing damages susceptible omega-6 fatty acids, they promote free radicals in your body.

Accordingly, your body should probably not use these broken fats as essential building blocks of your brain cells. Don't you think so?

Hence, for people who are intermittent fasting for health reasons, oat milk is not an option.

So, what about weight loss?

Besides the 7.5 grams of fat from canola oil, a glass

of oat milk has a staggering 16.5 grams of carbohydrates, of which 10 grams is table sugar.[60]

Thus, we no longer need to debate. That's the last nail in the coffin for oat milk during intermittent fasting.

Since even a shot of oat milk triggers a blood sugar and insulin spike, you better put it into the sink.

## Soy Milk

So, is soy milk another supposedly better alternative to milk while fasting?

One glass of soy milk has about 15.5 grams of carbohydrates, of which 10 grams is table sugar.[61]

As with oat milk, industrially produced omega-6 fatty acids predominate in this artificial drink.

Furthermore, the soy itself is one of the three most frequently genetically manipulated crops in the world. Accordingly, over 90% of the canola, corn, and soy harvest comes from genetically manipulated plants.

Why should your soy drink be non-GMO?

On the one hand, this is almost impossible to find out, and on the other hand, it is very unlikely.

Since the soy probably comes mainly from a foreign

country, the first processing steps happen somewhere, neither traceable nor regulated.

So what's the solution?

Eat real food! Industrially produced drinks mixed in a lab are harmful to your health – no matter what the commercials say.

However, a single shot of soy milk breaks the fast due to the high amount of carbohydrates.

With this in mind, if you need a milk substitute while eating due to an intolerance, go with unsweetened almond milk.

## Cocoa

Although a bit of cocoa powder is fine, you should pay attention to the amount.

Since the cocoa powder is made from the whole cocoa bean, it contains carbohydrates, protein, and fat. Therefore, more than a teaspoon of cocoa powder will break the fast.

There are two things to pay attention to with cocoa powder:

- It must be unsweetened
- Ideally, it is degreased too

Thus, a little cocoa powder moves in the gray area during the fasting period.

## Cinnamon

Cinnamon is okay as an additive. Moreover, it is a proven remedy against appetite and cravings. Therefore, it is welcome in our coffee during intermittent fasting.

Furthermore, cinnamon can even help to reduce insulin resistance. For example, the one you get due to lack of sleep.

Nevertheless, it is also true here that more significant amounts in coffee can impair autophagy.

## Nutmeg

Just like cinnamon, a little nutmeg can help against an acute appetite. Nevertheless, avoid excessive amounts as they can cause side effects.

## Bulletproof Coffee

The essential aspect of any Bulletproof Coffee is the addition of high-quality fat. Therefore, Bulletproof Coffee is not an ordinary coffee with milk.

It is a keto-friendly coffee drink that is also popular among intermittent fasting enthusiasts.

Additionally, many athletes or professional high performers also love Bulletproof Coffee. They all use keto coffee to get an energy boost from quickly metabolizable fat.

They leverage the drink to complete tasks more efficiently and quickly. Because this power drink helps you feel satiated and more focused, it's a staple in ketogenic kitchens and known to help with intermittent fasting.

The classic Bulletproof Coffee recipe includes black coffee and two essential ingredients:

- Fast-metabolizable MCT oil or coconut oil
- High-quality grass-fed butter or ghee

Although Bulletproof Coffee is repeatedly declared to be fasting-safe, it is not.

This fatty keto coffee may not cause insulin levels to skyrocket, but it does provide the body with plenty of fat.

So it doesn't stop ketosis, but as we know, the nutrient sensor AMPK responds to fat as well. Therefore, Bulletproof Coffee impairs autophagy.

Since it counteracts hunger, fasting beginners also use it as a tool to get used to intermittent fasting while lasting longer.

But which ingredients make Bulletproof Coffee unsuitable as a beverage during fasting periods?

## Coconut and MCT Oil

MCT stands for *medium-chain triglycerides* or medium-chain fatty acids.

Since it is derived from coconut oil but contains a much higher concentration of MCTs, MCT oil is effectively the powerful brother of coconut oil.

Because high-quality MCT oils can consist of caprylic acid, which is only eight carbon atoms long, they can be metabolized more efficiently than coconut oil.

Does coffee break the fast with this pure fat?

Although pure fats usually have many calories, they do not affect blood sugar. Nevertheless, it is a meal. And eating affects insulin levels.

However, in the case of pure fat, this happens only indirectly and minimally.

Therefore, technically, any fat breaks a fast. Hence, because of Bulletproof Coffee, you will burn less fat during the fasting period. Nonetheless, the impairment is minimal.

If you can initially get by with black coffee for only 12 hours, but with a few teaspoons of coconut oil in your coffee, you can last 18 hours, then the drawbacks of adding fat are probably justifiable.

Nonetheless, with 16/8 intermittent fasting, you won't need fat after a few days to extend the fast.

Ultimately, you'll want to burn your body fat instead.

## Butter and Ghee

Grass-fed butter gives classic Bulletproof Coffee a creamy consistency. It also contains high-quality fats that increase satiety and energy level.

Furthermore, grass-fed butter provides helpful nutrients such as vitamin A, beta-carotene, butyrates, or conjugated linoleic acid.

If you are looking for an allergy-friendly, shelf-stable option with almost no lactose, grass-fed ghee is your answer.

Butter, like coconut oil, ghee breaks a fast but should not significantly affect autophagy.

Although the intake of proteins interrupts this self-cleaning mechanism of the body, the amount in butter is negligible.

Ghee is even safer, as it is ultra-clarified butter without any lactose and protein.

## Tea

Green tea is probably the drink that has proved to be most effective in intermittent fasting over the decades. Moreover, besides water, tea is the most popular beverage in the world.

Meanwhile, only coffee can contest this title. Like coffee, a cup of tea has about 2.5 calories – both with[62] and without caffeine[63].

Nevertheless, many experts agree that this minimal amount of macronutrients in tea is negligible.

As with coffee, studies on green tea suggest that it induces rather than prevents autophagy.[64]

Furthermore, all pure varieties of natural tea are suitable for intermittent fasting. The degree of fermentation of the tea plant "Camellia Sinensis" determines the name of the tea:

- Unfermented – white tea
- Minimally fermented – green tea
- Partially fermented – oolong tea
- Fully fermented – black tea

Although all these teas are suitable, green tea provides the best properties for intermittent fasting due to its many active compounds[65,66,67]:

- Regulates blood sugar and prevents diabetes
- Boosts the metabolism
- Helps with fat burning
- Prevents cardiovascular diseases and cancer

Furthermore, real tea curbs the appetite, so it has already helped many people when fasting.

However, you should be careful with tea from coffee shops, which in most cases contain a lot of sugar[68] or at least sweeteners.

## Fruit Tea

Although fruit teas are prevalent here in Central Europe, they are often big surprises. You usually cannot be sure what is inside.

Besides regular dried fruits, candied fruits often hide in fruit tea. And their sugar content may break a fast.

Accordingly, the variance in fruit tea is significant.[69] Like green tea, it can contain almost none, just too many for intermittent fasting or a vast amount of hidden carbohydrates.

Therefore, as with food purchases, the basic rule is: read the label carefully and avoid any suspicious contents.

If you want to be on the safe side, do not drink fruit tea during fasting.

## Herbal Tea

Strictly speaking, herbal tea is not tea since it does not contain any constituents of the tea plant.

Nevertheless, it performs better than fruit tea since it does not necessarily contain dried fruit.

For example, the nutrient profile of pure chamomile tea hardly differs from black tea. Just like regular tea, chamomile tea has about 2.5 calories per cup and has traces of micronutrients.[70]

Many other pure herbal tea blends are also very similar to this composition.[71]

Therefore, pure herbal tea from the tea store or health food store is suitable for fasting. However, as with fruit tea, always check the ingredients and, if in doubt, refrain from buying it.

## Ginger and Chai Tea

In a broader sense, ginger and chai tea are pretty similar to regular herbal tea. If you can get the straight dried herbs in a tee specialty shop, you can drink the brewed tea during intermittent fasting.

Please keep your hands off instant mixes and chai from coffee shop chains, as they almost always contain additives that will break your fast.

If you are lucky, you can even get straight chai or ginger tea in grocery stores, but always check labels before purchasing.

However, it's not that easy to get it straight since most people drink chai as a latte. If the label says chai latte, it's going to break your fast anyway.

On the other hand, ginger tea brewed with nothing else than freshly chopped ginger root and hot water should be fine, as long as you don't eat the pieces.

## Tea With Milk

As we have since learned, even a shot of milk interferes with intermittent fasting after it causes blood sugar and insulin levels to spike.

If milk is low in fat, the spikes are even more significant. Just as in coffee, milk in tea is a no-go during fasting.

After both creamer and plant-based milk drinks are highly processed, they are also not suitable for fasting due to their ingredients.

Unfortunately, I have to disappoint the advocates of drinking tea the British way at this point. Only unsweetened almond milk moves in the gray area and will not necessarily break the fast with a splash in the tea.

In parallel with milk, we haven't yet looked at the second big question concerning hot beverages.

Are sweeteners allowed during intermittent fasting?

## Sweeteners

Sweet taste is a much-discussed topic in intermittent fasting and other dietary interventions. On the one hand, it isn't easy to entirely cut out the sweet taste, and on the other hand, it promotes cravings.

Most sugar-free sweeteners have zero protein, carbohydrates, and calories. Therefore, they do not raise blood sugar levels. But is the math that simple?

No. Unfortunately, people often forget that both intermittent fasting and most low-carb diets have one common goal. They aim to lower insulin levels, thereby allowing the body to tap into stored fat for energy.

The storage hormone insulin prevents the body from breaking down body fat and using it for energy. Consequently, a significant increase in insulin levels not only breaks the fast but also stops ketosis.

Unfortunately, many health websites have not done their homework in this regard.

As endocrinologist and fasting pioneer Dr. Jason Fung correctly points out, it doesn't matter if food raises blood sugar levels as long as it elevates insulin levels.[72]

And we will now take a closer look at to which sweeteners this effect applies.

## Honey

Honey still enjoys great popularity, especially in tea.

Nevertheless, the sweetener consists of over 80% sugar.[73] The fact that honey is natural does not help much. The table sugar from sugar beets is *natural* in the same way.

Consequently, tea with honey is not allowed during intermittent fasting.

Due to the considerable fructose content, honey, like conventional sugar, is not suitable for weight loss since this liver toxin promotes insulin resistance, type 2 diabetes, and fatty liver disease.

In short, "natural" does not always equal "healthy."

## Sugar

We have already talked enough about sugar to know that it breaks the fast.

After it already raises blood sugar, it's off the table. The high-calorie cocktail of glucose and fructose breaks any fast.

For this reason, it has no place in hot beverages while fasting. Instead, we should take a closer look at common sugar substitutes as potential alternatives.

## Sugar Alcohol

Unlike many other sweeteners, sugar alcohols are not calorie-free. Instead, they are dietary fibers, which are also usually labeled as such on the packaging.

Since the human body cannot properly digest these anti-nutrients, most of them are excreted. However, intestinal bacteria can consume them to a small extent.

For this reason, about 90% of the sugar alcohol consumed leaves the body unchanged.[74]

Xylitol is the most widely used sugar alcohol. It is also better known under a specific brand name in most countries.

However, xylitol is not non-nutritive. In addition, it triggers a small but significant increase in blood sugar levels.

After this stimulates digestion, xylitol can break a fast.[75]

In contrast, erythritol, another sugar alcohol, does not seem to have this effect. Besides, no significant increase in glucose and insulin levels has been observed with erythritol over a more extended period after ingestion.[76]

For this reason, it seems to be the best choice among sweeteners so far. However, after few researchers have looked into erythritol, I handle it in a gray area during fasting.

Still, I would only use this sweetener occasionally, as

it can cause addiction. Moreover, a strengthened craving for sweets will not be beneficial for weight loss efforts.

Both sweeteners made from sugar alcohols are marketed to us as *natural* sugar substitutes. However, xylitol, the supposed birch sugar, is not usually obtained from birch wood but straw or corncob residues.

Erythritol is also industrially produced from carbohydrates.

While xylitol-based sweeteners are produced in several steps using acids or alkalis, erythritol is obtained through microbial fermentation.

## Aspartame

As a decades-old ingredient in diet soda, aspartame or E951(additive declaration in Europe) is the best-known synthetic sweetener. This acquaintance of artificial sweeteners also includes acesulfame potassium in Zero drinks or sucralose.

They all provide no carbohydrates, protein, or calories. Nevertheless, studies show that even non-nutritive sweeteners can elevate insulin levels.

Furthermore, although aspartame, the classic sweetener in diet soda, does not affect blood sugar, it can sometimes raise insulin levels more severely than table sugar.

That's what a study comparing insulin levels after

consumption of sugar, stevia, and aspartame states. 30 minutes after consumption, the aspartame-sweetened food reached an absolute peak value that even table sugar could not reach.[77]

Accordingly, among a variety of other potential side effects, this sweetener prevents fat burning.

Aspartame contains large amounts of phenylalanine. Although it is a natural amino acid, it can be toxic in large doses.

The amino acid phenylalanine is chemically bound in aspartame and can thus be absorbed by the body quickly.

After it converts into so-called free methanol under higher temperatures, the phenylalanine in aspartame is of concern.

Once it is in this state, methanol can easily convert to formaldehyde.

Formaldehyde is a carcinogen (cancer-causing agent) that can cross the blood-brain barrier, a filter made of capillaries that carry blood to the brain and spinal cord.

Therefore, the researchers conclude that aspartame consumption may be harmful due to its contribution to the formation of formaldehyde adducts.[78]

The synthetically produced aspartame can therefore not be a safe option in interval fasting or in general.

## Acesulfame Potassium

The more heat-resistant sweetener acesulfame potassium with the E-number 950 is also used in commercially available beverages. You can find in particular in zero- and zero-sugar drinks. In most cases, a combination of aspartame and acesulfame potassium is used in these beverages.

Although acesulfame K is non-nutritive and sugar-free, it can stimulate insulin secretion.

In this context, researchers have even found that acesulfame potassium increases insulin levels to the same extent as the same amount of glucose.[79]

For this reason, „sugar-free" does not automatically mean „fasting-safe. " Not to mention that such a sweetener can generally be no help in losing weight.

## Sucralose

The third synthetic sweetener that the food industry uses a lot is sucralose.

You might better know sucralose by the name of a sweetener brand sold in sugar-like yellow packets. In the European Union, you'll also find it among the ingredients by the E-number 955.

As the name suggests, sucralose is related to sugar, yet it is non-nutritive.

Manufacturers produce it by the chlorination of sucrose. In short, they add chlorine atoms to regular sugar in a chemistry lab.

For this reason, unlike sugar, our bodies can no longer digest sucralose properly. Therefore, the sweetener is said to have both zero calories and zero net carbohydrates.

In addition, sucralose is about 600 times sweeter than regular sugar.[80]

A study published in the journal *Diabetes Care* compared drinking pure water with water sweetened with sucralose.

The oral intake of the sucralose drink increased the insulin levels of the test persons by up to 50 percent.[81]

Hence, the synthetic sweetener has a significant effect on insulin production.

Can plant-based sweeteners, therefore, perform better in comparison?

## Stevia

People hugely praise stevia since the sweetener is extracted from a plant, is sugar- and calorie-free.

Based on a well-known study, many marketers and writers claimed that stevia does not affect blood sugar or insulin levels.

Table sugar indeed causes higher glucose and insulin spikes immediately after consumption.

But even this much-cited study shows that the values change after about 90 minutes. From this point on, blood glucose and insulin levels are higher after consuming stevia than after consuming sugar.[82]

In contrast to this study, a more recent study compared the effects of these sweeteners for three hours instead of two.

Moreover, the subjects of this study consumed sweetened beverages, not sweetened meals. The researchers found no differences between table sugar and stevia on average over three hours.

Although sugar initially caused higher responses, the insulin production initiated by stevia was able to catch up throughout the experiment and adjust insulin levels overall.

It is also astonishing that blood glucose also increased. Ultimately, there was no difference on average between sugar and stevia for this value either.[83]

But it gets even more interesting, as another study says that steviol glycosides stimulate insulin secretion directly in the pancreas.[84]

Moreover, researchers have recently studied their molecular structure and found that steviol glycosides are confusingly similar to insulin.[85]

Therefore, they may bind to insulin receptors. Thus, stevia is not a safe choice and can break an intermittent fast.

## Agave Syrup

*Natural* sweeteners such as stevia or agave syrup are industrially processed, just like table sugar. Like sugar, they are refined from a plant source. The sugar beet is also a plant and, therefore, just as natural.

Unfortunately, these facts tend to get lost in the hymns of numerous marketing campaigns.

Nevertheless, we cannot directly compare agave syrup to stevia. While stevia is sugar-free and non-nutritive, agave syrup is a high-calorie carbohydrate bomb that breaks any fast.

It's also pure poison to the liver with up to 97% fructose content, making it diabetes in liquid form.

If you care about your health, you should avoid agave syrup as much as possible.

## Monk Fruit

Monk fruit has a similar effect to stevia. Like stevia or even aspartame, monk fruit extract is extremely sweet and gives beverages about 200 times the sweetness of sugar.

Also, it performed almost the same as stevia in a recent study.

For three hours after ingestion, the scientist did not find a significant difference in blood glucose and insulin concentrations on average between beverages sweetened with monk fruit extract and those sweetened with sugar.[86]

But there is even better evidence. One study found that monk fruit extract stimulates insulin production in the beta cells of the pancreas.

The researchers showed that mogroside V, which was isolated from the fruit, significantly increases insulin secretion.[87]

Although monk fruit extract might be one of the better alternatives, I still wouldn't use it every day. During fasting periods, it is not a safe choice either.

Also, according to studies, extreme sweetness promotes appetite and cravings, which is not known to help with weight loss.[88]

Although monk fruit extract or stevia may be acceptable in desserts on special occasions, they are not the miracle cures they are sold to us to be.

Anyone who has the goal of sustainable weight loss better crosses these natural sweeteners off the shopping list as well.

In addition, beverages sweetened with monk fruit extract have the potential to break your fast.

# Diet Soda

Light and zero drinks seem to be a legitimate alternative to traditional soda pop. Among their ingredients are no carbohydrates, proteins, and, ultimately, calories.

But as we know by now, sweeteners are a complex issue that relatively few people have had a chance to grapple with.

To examine diet drinks in terms of whether they are allowed during intermittent fasting, we need to know which sweeteners are inside.

Fortunately, in most cases, you can already guess the sweetener from the generic name of the drink.

## Diet Beverages

For a good reason, aspartame is probably the most common sweetener since the world's largest beverage manufacturers have been using it in diet drinks for decades.

Although calorie-free aspartame does not affect blood sugar levels, it sometimes elevates insulin more than table sugar.[89]

Therefore, the classic diet soda sweetener prevents not only autophagy but also fat burning.

Against this background, it is probably no coincidence that people who devour vast diet drinks are often particularly overweight.

Many people are not overweight despite drinking diet soda, but rather precisely because of their consumption.

## Zero Beverages

Although zero drinks vary in composition, they almost always contain the synthetic sweeteners aspartame and acesulfame potassium.

Apart from aspartame, the heat-stable sweetener acesulfame potassium in Zero drinks increases insulin levels to the same extent as glucose.[90]

Thus, these drinks are not a suitable choice during intermittent fasting and weight loss in general.

Moreover, the calorie-free sweeteners stimulate cravings in the brain and are, on balance, the greater evil than regular soda pop.[91]

Accordingly, researchers have found that consuming zero and diet beverages instead of regular soft drinks does not achieve the desired calorie reduction due to increased appetite.[92]

## Green Beverages

Stevia is the natural sweetener of the moment. That's why you can also find it in new product lines from beverage manufacturers.

Nevertheless, like table sugar, it is extracted from a plant and refined through complex processes. For this reason, some experts now classify stevia as an artificial sweetener.

Besides the fact that stevia-based sweeteners also increase glucose and insulin levels in the blood, there are other concerns about green drinks.

As a recent study shows, stevia alters the composition of the gut microbiome.[93]

Thus, it becomes clearer that stevia and green drinks are not suitable for intermittent fasting. Especially during fasting, gut health should be a priority.

## Energy and Sports Drinks

Regular energy drinks contain sugar. Thus, it would be best if you did not drink them during intermittent fasting either.

But also energy and sports drinks are now produced in all possible variants.

## Sugarfree Energy Drinks

Just like many zero or diet drinks, sugar-free energy drinks often contain aspartame and acesulfame potassium.

Since even sugar-free energy drinks contain artificial sweeteners, which significantly affect intermittent fasting, these drinks do not suit it.

## Zero Sports Drinks

Even if enrichment with electrolytes and vitamins sounds attractive at first glance, sugar-free sports drinks are not suitable for fasting.

For example, sports drinks from major manufacturers often contain sucralose in addition to acesulfame potassium. Studies have shown that just one packet of this sweetener can be enough to make a difference.

According to studies, one packet of this sweetener can be enough to wipe out 50 percent of healthy intestinal flora.[94]

In addition, sucralose anyway increases insulin levels and breaks fasting.[95]

## BCAA Drinks

Recently, amino acids have increasingly found their way into beverages. In addition to sports drinks, manufacturers of energy drinks have also recently started to use them.

But what is the primary purpose of *branched-chain amino acids (BCAAs)* in fitness drinks?

It's growth. That's why BCAA drinks stimulate the primary pathway for muscle growth in the human body, mTOR.

Therefore, drinking amino acid-enriched drinks switch off maintenance mode and turn on growth mode in the human body.

As we have already heard, mTOR is our body's primary nutrient sensor that turns off autophagy. In short, BCAA drinks are, therefore, the exact opposite of fasting-safe drinks.

For this reason, you should avoid them during intermittent fasting.

## Protein Shakes

Until the 1990s, scientists did not know that protein also can stimulate insulin secretion.[96]

For this reason, the first low-carb diets, such as the Atkins diet, were doomed to fail. The fact that the keto diet is based on this relatively new knowledge explains its popularity today.

Nevertheless, protein shakes still enjoy the image of weight loss drinks. However, hardly any beverage can stimulate insulin and mTOR like a protein shake with isolated whey protein.

Not only do protein shakes break a fast, but they also directly inhibit autophagy, which aims to reduce harmful protein accumulations, such as in the brain.[97]

Thus, autophagy counteracts our modern diseases characterized by too many proteins in the body supplied without need. These range from dementia to cardiovascular disease to cancer.

However, that does not mean proteins are negligible for muscle building, but their intake should fit the extent of training.

And at the end of the day, even with proteins, natural foods that are not highly processed are better.

## Collagen Protein

Intermittent fasting and keto enthusiasts love collagen in their drinks, such as in Bulletproof Coffee.

They have a good reason to do so since collagen is an essential building block for muscles, joints, skin, and hair.

Nevertheless, collagen powder is an isolated protein as well. On the one hand, protein activates the anabolic mTOR pathway for muscle building, and on the other hand, it thus inhibits autophagy.

Therefore, collagen can benefit muscle gain, fat burning, and satiety but breaks a fast.

## Exogenous Ketones

The ketogenic diet enjoys great popularity because of its weight-loss effectiveness and variety of health benefits.

With this in mind, people mix ketone supplements into their beverages to increase those benefits and athletic performance.

However, since our body makes ketones from fat, it is little wonder that exogenously supplied ketones also consist mainly of fat.[98]

Therefore, they are a meal and energy source that the body uses before resorting to body fat.

Just like a Bulletproof Coffee with considerable fat content, exogenous ketones in drinks, therefore, break the fast.

## Alcoholic Beverages

Because its effect is more intense on an empty stomach, you should not drink alcohol during intermittent fasting.

Moreover, alcohol is a source of calories that breaks a fast anyway.

Alcohol is also not a great idea during the eating window. Cocktails, mixed drinks, and especially beer are full of carbohydrates, stimulate insulin and appetite.

The exception is red wine, which can be drunk about glass size with dinner.[99]

According to scientific opinion, just this amount reveals health benefits, as the small amount of alcohol does not have a negative effect.[100]

Furthermore, red wine positively affects blood pressure, glucose, and insulin levels.[101]

If you choose a dry red wine like Pinot Noir with about 2.3 grams of carbohydrates per 100 milliliters, it can positively affect insulin sensitivity.[102]

The exciting thing about red wine is its parallels to green tea. Like tea, red wine contains various bioactive components that can provide a range of health benefits.

These are natural antioxidants, so-called polyphenols. One of the most potent polyphenols is found exclusively in red wine.

The polyphenol resveratrol comes from the grape skin. Unlike red wine, however, white wine has the skin removed before fermentation. Therefore, white wine does not contain resveratrol.

The most significant advantage of resveratrol is that

it is one of the few substances that, according to current findings, can promote autophagy by inhibiting the mTOR pathway.[103]

Although red wine is taboo during the fasting period, a glass with dinner can support the health goals of fasting.

# Training Wheels

To me, training wheels are beverages that make it easier for your body to get used to the changes in metabolism caused by intermittent fasting.

On the one hand, these can be special drinks, and on the other hand, natural additions to the most popular fasting beverages.

In the course of evaluating various drinks, we have already become acquainted with most of these starting aids for intermittent fasting:

- Lemon, lime, or Himalayan salt in water.

- Cinnamon, cocoa powder, or nutmeg in a coffee

- Bulletproof coffee as a popular energy booster

- Butter, ghee, MCT, coconut oil, or almond milk in coffee and tea

Against this background, we can derive the following tasks of our training wheels:

- Avoidance of cravings
- Reduction of physical side effects
- Promotion of long-term satiety
- Option as an additional energy source
- Preservation of taste diversity

Depending on how people have been eating before, it can take three to six weeks for the metabolism to adjust to intermittent fasting and burn fat for energy.

Over this period, it is okay to use the tools explained. After that, it should be easy to get by without starting aids and not unnecessarily limit the effects of intermittent fasting.

However, we have to take a detailed look at some of the best beverages that have proven themselves as potential training wheels.

## Bone Broth

Homemade bone broth from beef, pork, or chicken bones, not only tastes great but also has properties that help with fasting:

- It provides electrolytes,
- Is easily digestible,
- Helps absorb nutrients due to natural fat.

But here is already the crux of the matter. Broth contains enough fat to activate AMPK and break the fast.

Therefore, bone broth is instead one of the best options after breaking the fast.

Since magnesium, potassium, calcium, and sodium are in bone broth, it can replenish the electrolytes flushed out.

Accordingly, bone broth is used as an electrolyte donor during fasting, for example, during therapeutic fasting for days or weeks. Therefore, it represents a starting aid for beginners, helping to familiarize the body with intermittent fasting.

In the process, bone broth also prevents physical side effects of the metabolic change due to electrolyte loss.


## Pickle Juice

Like bone broth, sugar-free pickle water has helped many people during fasting. While broth is a comprehensive electrolyte donor, the cucumber water provides salt in particular.

That's why you should drink it during intermittent or therapeutic fasting when acute symptoms of the keto-flu like headache or dizziness appear.

Nevertheless, pickle juice, like bone broth, should be a starting aid you can discard once the body has become accustomed to intermittent fasting.

## Apple Cider Vinegar

Apple cider vinegar helps people who are predominantly used to digesting carbohydrates and proteins to more easily incorporate healthy fats into their diet for nutrient absorption.

Moreover, drinking apple cider vinegar supports intermittent fasting due to the following benefits:

- Reduces blood sugar and promotes insulin sensitivity[104]

- Increases satiety and reduces the risk of overeating[105]

- Stimulates fat burning and helps weight loss[106]

- Releases stomach and intestine neutralizing hormones and ions[107]

- Prevents heartburn and acid reflux

For these reasons, followers of low-carb diets such as the keto diet swear by apple cider vinegar.

Even fasting beginners use apple cider vinegar diluted with water all the time. From a purely technical standpoint, an apple cider vinegar drink could affect autophagy, but the tiny amounts of micro and macronutrients are negligible, similar to coffee.[108]

Nonetheless, it represents a tool like broth if you want to go over new distances during fasting. Furthermore, apple cider vinegar is also a prime beverage for breaking a fast due to its positive effects on blood sugar and digestion.

# Conclusion

Besides all the success stories about intermittent fasting, hardly anyone speaks plainly about how it works in our bodies.

In the end, this way of eating is not as simple as one would like to believe. To find out what to drink during a fasting period requires knowledge of essential processes in the body.

For this reason, this book aims at deriving comprehensible measures regarding questions nobody could answer so far. Drinking is still the topic where most mistakes are made during intermittent fasting.

If there's one thing we've learned, it's that details make a difference, such as with sweeteners.

Activation and inhibition of autophagy are essential

factors in achieving health benefits from intermittent fasting.

In this context, there are still many nuances of our body that have not been explored. What we can do at this point, however, is make a clear summary of the following drinks that are safe for fasting:

- Water (with a squeeze of lemon)
- Mineral water
- Black coffee
- Black decaffeinated coffee
- White tea
- Green tea
- Oolong tea
- Black tea
- Herbal tea (check ingredients)

We can also summarize that these beverages have to be consumed without milk, sugar, or sweeteners.

What you can drink during intermittent fasting always depends on your individual goals. If you practice it for weight loss, then you are on the right track with this list.

Research is not yet in complete agreement regarding extended autophagy fasting for disease prevention and longevity.

Although numerous animal studies suggest that coffee and green tea support autophagy, the truth is that we don't know for sure.

Nevertheless, green tea has been shown to induce autophagy in human cells. However, these cells were previously implanted in mice.[109]

Since there is no corresponding data for humans yet, autophagy fasting is often practiced as pure water fasting, limiting your nutrient intake to natural salt, sole water (see recipes), or mineral water.

Since there is always a certain basic level of auto-phagy in the body, it is not immediately switched off from 100% to 0%.

Accordingly, your fasting goals are essential. Training wheels can be helpful if you are just starting and want to improve fat burning in particular.

However, if your declared goal is a comprehensive detox of your body, water is your best companion.

Within the framework of this book, I have tried to answer all questions that arise in connection with beverages during intermittent fasting.

Nevertheless, one or the other new question will always come up.

For this reason, I offer my readers to get in touch with me via my blog if any questions remain unanswered.

This concept has already worked with hundreds of articles to help numerous readers with their unique questions.

# Recipes

After repeatedly coming across drinks, which can help beginners jump-start intermittent fasting, here are the appropriate recipes to prepare them.

## Bone Broth

- **4 lbs beef bones** (cut with marrow)
- **1 slice celeriac**
- **1 pcs leek**
- **2 pcs carrots**
- **1 pcs onion** (yellow)
- **2 pcs bay leaves**
- **1 tsp juniper berries**
- **1 tsp peppercorns**
- **2-3 tsp pink Himalayan salt**
- **145 oz water** (filtered, enough to cover the bones)
- **1-2 tbsp apple cider vinegar**

Peel the carrots, leek, and celery and cut them into coarse pieces. Then cut the onion in half, but do not peel it since the peel gives the soup a lovely color.

Now fry the onion halves briefly in the pot with the cut side down. Then add the rest of the vegetables and bones and fill the pot with water.

Add spices and apple cider vinegar, the acidity of which helps to extract collagen and minerals from the bones better.

Bring to a boil, then reduce to a simmer and cover. Simmer for 12 hours. The further it reduces, the more intense the flavor will be, and the more collagen will be extracted. Optionally, you can add water and get a thinner broth. Alternatively, you can use an Instant Pot as well.

Strain broth and enjoy or store.

*Makes 12 Cups*

# Bulletproof Coffee

- **2½ tbsp coffee** (freshly ground)
- **1-2 tbsp MCT oil** (or coconut oil)
- **1-2 tbsp grass-fed Ghee** (or Butter)

Brew a cup of coffee using 2 ½ tablespoons of freshly ground coffee beans.

Add one teaspoon to 2 tablespoons of MCT oil. Start with one teaspoon and work your way up to 1-2 tablespoons over several days.

Add 1-2 tablespoons of grass-fed butter or ghee.

Mix everything in a blender for 20-30 seconds until it looks like a creamy latte.

*Makes one cup*

# Apple Cider Vinegar Drink

- **One glass of water** (8oz)
- **1-2 tbsp apple cider vinegar**

Mix ingredients in a highball glass and serve cold.

*Makes one glass*

# Sole Water

- **1 cup Himalayan Pink Salt**
- **34 fl oz Water** (filtered)

Fill about 1/4 of the glass container with Himalayan salt.

Add the water until about two inches remain free at the top.

Place the lid on top and gently shake the container. Let the glass container sit overnight to allow the salt to dissolve.

If salt remains at the bottom of the jar the next day, the water has absorbed the maximum salt, and the sole is ready.

Otherwise, add salt to the water again and continue if no salt remains at the bottom the next day.

*Makes 34 fl oz*

# References

[1]Natalucci G, Riedl S, Gleiss A, Zidek T, Frisch H. Spontaneous 24-h ghrelin secretion pattern in fasting subjects: maintenance of a meal-related pattern. Eur J Endocrinol. 2005 Jun;152(6):845-50. doi: 10.1530/eje.1.01919. PubMed PMID: 15941923.

[2]Levine B, Klionsky DJ. Autophagy wins the 2016 Nobel Prize in Physiology or Medicine: Breakthroughs in baker's yeast fuel advances in biomedical research. Proc Natl Acad Sci U S A. 2017 Jan 10;114(2):201-205. doi: 10.1073/pnas.1619876114. Epub 2016 Dec 30. PubMed PMID: 28039434; PubMed Central PMCID: PMC5240711.

[3] Yang JS, Lu CC, Kuo SC, Hsu YM, Tsai SC, Chen SY, Chen YT, Lin YJ, Huang YC, Chen CJ, Lin WD, Liao WL, Lin WY, Liu YH, Sheu JC, Tsai FJ. Autophagy and its link to type II diabetes mellitus. Biomedicine (Taipei). 2017 Jun;7(2):8. doi: 10.1051/bmdcn/2017070201. Epub 2017 Jun 14. PubMed PMID: 28612706; PubMed Central PMCID: PMC5479440.

[4] Fung J. The Obesity Code: Unlocking the Secrets of Weight Loss. Vancouver: Greystone Books, 2016.

[5] Park J, Kwock CK, Yang YJ. The Effect of the Sodium to Potassium Ratio on Hypertension Prevalence: A Propensity Score Matching Approach. Nutrients. 2016 Aug 6;8(8). doi: 10.3390/nu8080482. PubMed PMID: 27509520; PubMed Central PMCID: PMC4997395.

[6] Fung J. The Obesity Code: Unlocking the Secrets of Weight Loss. Vancouver: Greystone Books, 2016.

[7] Sakuyama H, Katoh M, Wakabayashi H, Zulli A, Kruzliak P, Uehara Y. Influence of gestational salt restriction in fetal growth and in development of diseases in adulthood. J Biomed Sci. 2016 Jan 20;23:12. doi: 10.1186/s12929-016-0233-8. Review. PubMed PMID: 26787358; PubMed Central PMCID: PMC4719732.

[8]Ho KY, Veldhuis JD, Johnson ML, Furlanetto R, Evans WS, Alberti KG, Thorner MO. Fasting enhances growth hormone secretion and amplifies the complex rhythms of growth hormone secretion in man. J Clin Invest. 1988 Apr;81(4):968-75. doi: 10.1172/JCI113450. PubMed PMID: 3127426; PubMed Central PMCID: PMC329619.

[9]Meijssen S, Cabezas MC, Ballieux CG, Derksen RJ, Bilecen S, Erkelens DW. Insulin mediated inhibition of hormone sensitive lipase activity in vivo in relation to endogenous catecholamines in healthy subjects. J Clin Endocrinol Metab. 2001 Sep;86(9):4193-7. doi: 10.1210/jcem.86.9.7794. PubMed PMID: 11549649.

[10]Kong LC, Wuillemin PH, Bastard JP, Sokolovska N, Gougis S, Fellahi S, Darakhshan F, Bonnefont-Rousselot D, Bittar R, Doré J, Zucker JD, Clément K, Rizkalla S. Insulin resistance and inflammation predict kinetic body weight changes in response to dietary weight loss and maintenance in overweight and obese subjects by using a Bayesian network approach. Am J Clin Nutr. 2013 Dec;98(6):1385-94. doi: 10.3945/ajcn.113.058099. Epub 2013 Oct 30. PubMed PMID: 24172304.

[11]Lustig RH. The neuroendocrinology of childhood obesity. Pediatr Clin North Am. 2001 Aug;48(4):909-30. doi: 10.1016/s0031-3955(05)70348-5. Review. PubMed PMID: 11494643.

[12]Levine B, Klionsky DJ. Autophagy wins the 2016 Nobel Prize in Physiology or Medicine: Breakthroughs in baker's yeast fuel advances in biomedical research. Proc Natl Acad Sci U S A. 2017 Jan 10;114(2):201-205. doi: 10.1073/pnas.1619876114. Epub 2016 Dec 30. PubMed PMID: 28039434; PubMed Central PMCID: PMC5240711.

[13]Bagherniya M, Butler AE, Barreto GE, Sahebkar A. The effect of fasting or calorie restriction on autophagy induction: A review of the literature. Ageing Res Rev. 2018 Nov;47:183-197. doi: 10.1016/j.arr.2018.08.004. Epub 2018 Aug 30. Review. PubMed PMID: 30172870.

[14]Raefsky SM, Mattson MP. Adaptive responses of neuronal mitochondria to bioenergetic challenges: Roles in neuroplasticity and disease resistance. Free Radic Biol Med. 2017 Jan;102:203-216. doi: 10.1016/j.freeradbiomed.2016.11.045. Epub 2016 Nov 29. Review. PubMed PMID: 27908782; PubMed Central PMCID: PMC5209274.

[15]Jiao J, Demontis F. Skeletal muscle autophagy and its role in sarcopenia and organismal aging. Curr Opin Pharmacol. 2017 Jun;34:1-6. doi: 10.1016/j.coph.2017.03.009. Epub 2017 Apr 10. Review. PubMed PMID: 28407519.

[16]Sasaki Y, Ikeda Y, Iwabayashi M, Akasaki Y, Ohishi M. The Impact of Autophagy on Cardiovascular Senescence and Diseases. Int Heart J. 2017 Oct 21;58(5):666-673. doi: 10.1536/ihj.17-246. Epub 2017 Sep 30. Review. PubMed PMID: 28966332.

[17]Nakamura S, Yoshimori T. Autophagy and Longevity. Mol Cells. 2018 Jan 31;41(1):65-72. doi: 10.14348/molcells.2018.2333. Epub 2018 Jan 23. Review. PubMed PMID: 29370695; PubMed Central PMCID: PMC5792715.

[18]Yang JS, Lu CC, Kuo SC, Hsu YM, Tsai SC, Chen SY, Chen YT, Lin YJ, Huang YC, Chen CJ, Lin WD, Liao WL, Lin WY, Liu YH, Sheu JC, Tsai FJ. Autophagy and its link to type II diabetes mellitus. Biomedicine (Taipei). 2017 Jun;7(2):8. doi: 10.1051/bmdcn/2017070201. Epub 2017 Jun 14. PubMed PMID: 28612706; PubMed Central PMCID: PMC5479440.

[19]Sasaki Y, Ikeda Y, Iwabayashi M, Akasaki Y, Ohishi M. The Impact of Autophagy on Cardiovascular Senescence and Diseases. Int Heart J. 2017 Oct 21;58(5):666-673. doi: 10.1536/ihj.17-246. Epub 2017 Sep 30. Review. PubMed PMID: 28966332.

[20] Gelino S, Hansen M. Autophagy – An Emerging Anti-Aging Mechanism. J Clin Exp Pathol. 2012 Jul 12;Suppl 4. doi: 10.4172/2161-0681.s4-006. PubMed PMID: 23750326; PubMed Central PMCID: PMC3674854.

[21]Nakamura S, Yoshimori T. Autophagy and Longevity. Mol Cells. 2018 Jan 31;41(1):65-72. doi: 10.14348/molcells.2018.2333. Epub 2018 Jan 23. Review. PubMed PMID: 29370695; PubMed Central PMCID: PMC5792715.

[22] Catterson JH, Khericha M, Dyson MC, Vincent AJ, Callard R, Haveron SM, Rajasingam A, Ahmad M, Partridge L. Short-Term, Intermittent Fasting Induces Long-Lasting Gut Health and TOR-Independent Lifespan Extension. Curr Biol. 2018 Jun 4;28(11):1714-1724.e4. doi: 10.1016/j.cub.2018.04.015.Epub 2018 May 17. PubMed PMID: 29779873; PubMed Central PMCID: PMC5988561.

[23] Li X, Chen H, Guan Y, Li X, Lei L, Liu J, Yin L, Liu G, Wang Z. Acetic acid activates the AMP-activated protein kinase signaling pathway to regulate lipid metabolism in bovine hepatocytes. PLoS One. 2013;8(7):e67880. doi: 10.1371/journal.pone.0067880. Print 2013. PubMed PMID: 23861826; PubMed Central PMCID: PMC3701595.

[24] Raefsky SM, Mattson MP. Adaptive responses of neuronal mitochondria to bioenergetic challenges: Roles in neuroplasticity and disease resistance. Free Radic Biol Med. 2017 Jan;102:203-216. doi: 10.1016/j.freeradbiomed.2016.11.045. Epub 2016 Nov 29. Review. PubMed PMID: 27908782; PubMed Central PMCID: PMC5209274.

[25] Witte AV, Fobker M, Gellner R, Knecht S, Flöel A. Caloric restriction improves memory in elderly humans. Proc Natl Acad Sci U S A. 2009 Jan 27;106(4):1255-60. doi: 10.1073/pnas.0808587106. Epub 2009 Jan 26. PubMed PMID: 19171901; PubMed Central PMCID: PMC2633586.

[26]Lieberman HR, Caruso CM, Niro PJ, Adam GE, Kellogg MD, Nindl BC, Kramer FM. A double-blind, placebo-controlled test of 2 d of calorie deprivation: effects on cognition, activity, sleep, and interstitial glucose concentrations. Am J Clin Nutr. 2008 Sep;88(3):667-76. doi: 10.1093/ajcn/88.3.667. PubMed PMID: 18779282.

[27]DRENICK EJ, SWENDSEID ME, BLAHD WH, TUTTLE SG. PROLONGED STARVATION AS TREATMENT FOR SEVERE OBESITY. JAMA. 1964 Jan 11;187:100-5. doi: 10.1001/jama.1964.03060150024006. PubMed PMID: 14066725.

[28]Ho KY, Veldhuis JD, Johnson ML, Furlanetto R, Evans WS, Alberti KG, Thorner MO. Fasting enhances growth hormone secretion and amplifies the complex rhythms of growth hormone secretion in man. J Clin Invest. 1988 Apr;81(4):968-75. doi: 10.1172/JCI113450. PubMed PMID: 3127426; PubMed Central PMCID: PMC329619.

[29]Zauner C, Schneeweiss B, Kranz A, Madl C, Ratheiser K, Kramer L, Roth E, Schneider B, Lenz K. Resting energy expenditure in short-term starvation is increased as a result of an increase in serum norepinephrine. Am J Clin Nutr. 2000 Jun;71(6):1511-5. doi: 10.1093/ajcn/71.6.1511. PubMed PMID: 10837292.

[30]Rudman D, Feller AG, Nagraj HS, Gergans GA, Lalitha PY, Goldberg AF, Schlenker RA, Cohn L, Rudman IW, Mattson DE. Effects of human growth hormone in men over 60 years old. N Engl J Med. 1990 Jul 5;323(1):1-6. doi: 10.1056/NEJM199007053230101. PubMed PMID: 2355952.

[31]Ho KY, Veldhuis JD, Johnson ML, Furlanetto R, Evans WS, Alberti KG, Thorner MO. Fasting enhances growth hormone secretion and amplifies the complex rhythms of growth hormone secretion in man. J Clin Invest. 1988 Apr;81(4):968-75. doi: 10.1172/JCI113450. PubMed PMID: 3127426; PubMed Central PMCID: PMC329619.

[32]Paoli A, Bosco G, Camporesi EM, Mangar D. Ketosis, ketogenic diet and food intake control: a complex relationship. Front Psychol. 2015;6:27. doi: 10.3389/fpsyg.2015.00027. eCollection 2015. Review. PubMed PMID: 25698989; PubMed Central PMCID: PMC4313585.

[33]Hallböök T, Ji S, Maudsley S, Martin B. The effects of the ketogenic diet on behavior and cognition. Epilepsy Res. 2012 Jul;100(3):304-9. doi: 10.1016/j.eplepsyres.2011.04.017. Epub 2011 Aug 27. Review. PubMed PMID: 21872440; PubMed Central PMCID: PMC4112040.

[34]Catenacci VA, Pan Z, Ostendorf D, Brannon S, Gozansky WS, Mattson MP, Martin B, MacLean PS, Melanson EL, Troy Donahoo W. A randomized pilot study comparing zero-calorie alternate-day fasting to daily caloric restriction in adults with obesity. Obesity (Silver Spring). 2016 Sep;24(9):1874-83. doi: 10.1002/oby.21581. PubMed PMID: 27569118; PubMed Central PMCID: PMC5042570.

[35]Bray GA, Jablonski KA, Fujimoto WY, Barrett-Connor E, Haffner S, Hanson RL, Hill JO, Hubbard V, Kriska A, Stamm E, Pi-Sunyer FX. Relation of central adiposity and body mass index to the development of diabetes in the Diabetes Prevention Program. Am J Clin Nutr. 2008 May;87(5):1212-8. doi: 10.1093/ajcn/87.5.1212. PubMed PMID: 18469241; PubMed Central PMCID: PMC2517222.

[36]Jackson IM, McKiddie MT, Buchanan KD. Effect of fasting on glucose and insulin metabolism of obese patients. Lancet. 1969 Feb 8;1(7589):285-7. doi: 10.1016/s0140-6736(69)91039-3. PubMed PMID: 4178981.

[37]Catenacci VA, Pan Z, Ostendorf D, Brannon S, Gozansky WS, Mattson MP, Martin B, MacLean PS, Melanson EL, Troy Donahoo W. A randomized pilot study comparing zero-calorie alternate-day fasting to daily caloric restriction in adults with obesity. Obesity (Silver Spring). 2016 Sep;24(9):1874-83. doi: 10.1002/oby.21581. PubMed PMID: 27569118; PubMed Central PMCID: PMC5042570.

[38] Halberg N, Henriksen M, Söderhamn N, Stallknecht B, Ploug T, Schjerling P, Dela F. Effect of intermittent fasting and refeeding on insulin action in healthy men. J Appl Physiol (1985). 2005 Dec;99(6):2128-36. doi: 10.1152/japplphysiol.00683.2005. Epub 2005 Jul 28. PubMed PMID: 16051710.

[39] Ali AT. Polycystic ovary syndrome and metabolic syndrome. Ceska Gynekol. 2015 Aug;80(4):279-89. Review. PubMed PMID: 26265416.

[40] Nair PM, Khawale PG. Role of therapeutic fasting in women's health: An overview. J Midlife Health. 2016 Apr-Jun;7(2):61-4. doi: 10.4103/0976-7800.185325. Review. PubMed PMID: 27499591; PubMed Central PMCID: PMC4960941.

[41] Catterson JH, Khericha M, Dyson MC, Vincent AJ, Callard R, Haveron SM, Rajasingam A, Ahmad M, Partridge L. Short-Term, Intermittent Fasting Induces Long-Lasting Gut Health and TOR-Independent Lifespan Extension. Curr Biol. 2018 Jun 4;28(11):1714-1724.e4. doi: 10.1016/j.cub.2018.04.015. Epub 2018 May 17. PubMed PMID: 29779873; PubMed Central PMCID: PMC5988561.

[42] Stewart WK, Fleming LW. Features of a successful therapeutic fast of 382 days' duration. Postgrad Med J. 1973 Mar;49(569):203-9. doi: 10.1136/pgmj.49.569.203. PubMed PMID: 4803438; PubMed Central PMCID: PMC2495396.

[43] *The Self NutritionData method and system [Internet]. New York: Condé Nast; c2018 [cited 2021 Jan 29]. Available from: https://nutrition-data.self.com/facts/nut-and-seed-products/3115/2.*

[44] *Angulo P, Lindor KD. Non-alcoholic fatty liver disease. J Gastroenterol Hepatol. 2002 Feb;17 Suppl:S186-90. doi: 10.1046/j.1440-1746.17.s1.10.x. Review. PubMed PMID: 12000605.*

[45] *The Self NutritionData method and system [Internet]. New York: Condé Nast; c2018 [cited 2021 Jan 29]. Available from: https://nutrition-data.self.com/facts/vegetables-and-vegetable-products/2396/2.*

[46] *Pietrocola F, Malik SA, Mariño G, Vacchelli E, Senovilla L, Chaba K, Niso-Santano M, Maiuri MC, Madeo F, Kroemer G. Coffee induces autophagy in vivo. Cell Cycle. 2014;13(12):1987-94. doi: 10.4161/cc.28929. Epub 2014 Apr 25. PubMed PMID: 24769862; PubMed Central PMCID: PMC4111762.*

[47] *Icken D, Feller S, Engeli S, Mayr A, Müller A, Hilbert A, de Zwaan M. Caffeine intake is related to successful weight loss maintenance. Eur J Clin Nutr. 2016 Apr;70(4):532-4. doi: 10.1038/ejcn.2015.183. Epub 2015 Nov 11. PubMed PMID: 26554757.*

[48] *Greenberg JA, Geliebter A. Coffee, hunger, and peptide YY. J Am Coll Nutr. 2012 Jun;31(3):160-6. doi: 10.1080/07315724.2012.10720023. PubMed PMID: 23204152.*

[49] Acheson KJ, Zahorska-Markiewicz B, Pittet P, Anantharaman K, Jéquier E. Caffeine and coffee: their influence on metabolic rate and substrate utilization in normal weight and obese individuals. Am J Clin Nutr. 1980 May;33(5):989-97. doi: 10.1093/ajcn/33.5.989. PubMed PMID: 7369170.

[50] Vandenberghe C, St-Pierre V, Courchesne-Loyer A, Hennebelle M, Castellano CA, Cunnane SC. Caffeine intake increases plasma ketones: an acute metabolic study in humans. Can J Physiol Pharmacol. 2017 Apr;95(4):455-458. doi: 10.1139/cjpp-2016-0338. Epub 2016 Nov 25. PubMed PMID: 28177691.

[51] Merimee TJ, Tyson JE. Stabilization of plasma glucose during fasting; Normal variations in two separate studies. N Engl J Med. 1974 Dec 12;291(24):1275-8. doi: 10.1056/NEJM197412122912404. PubMed PMID: 4431434.

[52] Carlström M, Larsson SC. Coffee consumption and reduced risk of developing type 2 diabetes: a systematic review with meta-analysis. Nutr Rev. 2018 Jun 1;76(6):395-417. doi: 10.1093/nutrit/nuy014. PubMed PMID: 29590460.

[53] van Dam RM, Pasman WJ, Verhoef P. Effects of coffee consumption on fasting blood glucose and insulin concentrations: randomized controlled trials in healthy volunteers. Diabetes Care. 2004 Dec;27(12):2990-2. doi: 10.2337/diacare.27.12.2990. PubMed PMID: 15562223.

[54]Smits P, Pieters G, Thien T. The role of epinephrine in the circulatory effects of coffee. Clin Pharmacol Ther. 1986 Oct;40(4):431-7. doi: 10.1038/clpt.1986.203. PubMed PMID: 3530587.

[55]Sherwin RS, Saccà L. Effect of epinephrine on glucose metabolism in humans: contribution of the liver. Am J Physiol. 1984 Aug;247(2 Pt 1):E157-65. doi: 10.1152/ajpendo.1984.247.2.E157. PubMed PMID: 6380304.

[56]Greenberg JA, Geliebter A. Coffee, hunger, and peptide YY. J Am Coll Nutr. 2012 Jun;31(3):160-6. doi: 10.1080/07315724.2012.10720023. PubMed PMID: 23204152.

[57]Bagherniya M, Butler AE, Barreto GE, Sahebkar A. The effect of fasting or calorie restriction on autophagy induction: A review of the literature. Ageing Res Rev. 2018 Nov;47:183-197. doi: 10.1016/j.arr.2018.08.004. Epub 2018 Aug 30. Review. PubMed PMID: 30172870.

[58]Acheson KJ, Zahorska-Markiewicz B, Pittet P, Anantharaman K, Jéquier E. Caffeine and coffee: their influence on metabolic rate and substrate utilization in normal weight and obese individuals. Am J Clin Nutr. 1980 May;33(5):989-97. doi: 10.1093/ajcn/33.5.989. PubMed PMID: 7369170.

[59]Icken D, Feller S, Engeli S, Mayr A, Müller A, Hilbert A, de Zwaan M. Caffeine intake is related to successful weight loss maintenance. Eur J Clin Nutr. 2016 Apr;70(4):532-4. doi: 10.1038/ejcn.2015.183. Epub 2015 Nov 11. PubMed PMID: 26554757.

[60]*Eat This Much Inc [Internet]. California: Redondo Beach; c2018 [cited 2021 Jan 29]. Available from: https://nutritiondata.self.com/facts/vegetables-and-vegetable-products/2396/2.*

[61]*The Self NutritionData method and system [Internet]. New York: Condé Nast; c2018 [cited 2021 Jan 29]. Available from: https://nutrition-data.self.com/facts/legumes-and-legume-products/4387/2.*

[62]*The Self NutritionData method and system [Internet]. New York: Condé Nast; c2018 [cited 2021 Jan 29]. Available from: https://nutri-tiondata.self.com/facts/beverages/4019/2.*

[63]*The Self NutritionData method and system [Internet]. New York: Condé Nast; c2018 [cited 2021 Jan 29]. Available from: https://nutri-tiondata.self.com/facts/beverages/3965/2.*

[64]*Prasanth MI, Sivamaruthi BS, Chaiyasut C, Tencomnao T. A Review of the Role of Green Tea (Camellia sinensis) in Antiphotoaging, Stress Resistance, Neuroprotection, and Autophagy. Nutrients. 2019 Feb 23;11(2). doi: 10.3390/nu11020474. Review. PubMed PMID: 30813433; PubMed Central PMCID: PMC6412948.*

[65]*Crespy V, Williamson G. A review of the health effects of green tea catechins in in vivo animal models. J Nutr. 2004 Dec;134(12 Suppl):3431S-3440S. doi: 10.1093/jn/134.12.3431S. PMID: 15570050.*

[66] Hursel R, Westerterp-Plantenga MS. Catechin- and caffeine-rich teas for control of body weight in humans. Am J Clin Nutr. 2013 Dec;98(6 Suppl):1682S-1693S. doi: 10.3945/ajcn.113.058396. Epub 2013 Oct 30. PMID: 24172301.

[67] Dulloo AG, Seydoux J, Girardier L, Chantre P, Vandermander J. Green tea and thermogenesis: interactions between catechin-polyphenols, caffeine and sympathetic activity. Int J Obes Relat Metab Disord. 2000 Feb;24(2):252-8. doi: 10.1038/sj.ijo.0801101. PMID: 10702779.

[68] The Self NutritionData method and system [Internet]. New York: Condé Nast; c2018 [cited 2021 Jan 29]. Available from: https://nutritiondata.self.com/facts/foods-from-starbucks/9646/2.

[69] MyFitnessPal Inc [Internet]. California: San Francisco; c2021 [cited 2021 Jan 29]. Available from: https://www.myfitnesspal.com/nutrition-facts-calories/fruit-tea.

[70] The Self NutritionData method and system [Internet]. New York: Condé Nast; c2018 [cited 2021 Jan 29]. Available from: https://nutritiondata.self.com/facts/beverages/4020/2.

[71] The Self NutritionData method and system [Internet]. New York: Condé Nast; c2018 [cited 2021 Jan 29]. Available from: https://nutritiondata.self.com/facts/beverages/3979/2.

[72] Fung J. The Obesity Code: Unlocking the Secrets of Weight Loss. Vancouver: Greystone Books, 2016.

[73] *The Self NutritionData method and system [Internet]. New York: Condé Nast; c2018 [cited 2021 Jan 29]. Available from: https://nutritiondata.self.com/facts/sweets/5568/2.*

[74] *Noda K, Nakayama K, Oku T. Serum glucose and insulin levels and erythritol balance after oral administration of erythritol in healthy subjects. Eur J Clin Nutr. 1994 Apr;48(4):286-92. PubMed PMID: 8039489.*

[75] *Natah SS, Hussien KR, Tuominen JA, Koivisto VA. Metabolic response to lactitol and xylitol in healthy men. Am J Clin Nutr. 1997 Apr;65(4):947-50. doi: 10.1093/ajcn/65.4.947. PubMed PMID: 9094877.*

[76] *Bornet FR, Blayo A, Dauchy F, Slama G. Plasma and urine kinetics of erythritol after oral ingestion by healthy humans. Regul Toxicol Pharmacol. 1996 Oct;24(2 Pt 2):S280-5. doi: 10.1006/rtph.1996.0109. PubMed PMID: 8933644.*

[77] *Anton SD, Martin CK, Han H, Coulon S, Cefalu WT, Geiselman P, Williamson DA. Effects of stevia, aspartame, and sucrose on food intake, satiety, and postprandial glucose and insulin levels. Appetite. 2010 Aug;55(1):37-43. doi: 10.1016/j.appet.2010.03.009. Epub 2010 Mar 18. PubMed PMID: 20303371; PubMed Central PMCID: PMC2900484.*

[78] Trocho C, Pardo R, Rafecas I, Virgili J, Remesar X, Fernández-López JA, Alemany M. Formaldehyde derived from dietary aspartame binds to tissue components in vivo. Life Sci. 1998;63(5):337-49. doi: 10.1016/s0024-3205(98)00282-3. PubMed PMID: 9714421.

[79] Liang Y, Steinbach G, Maier V, Pfeiffer EF. The effect of artificial sweetener on insulin secretion. 1. The effect of acesulfame K on insulin secretion in the rat (studies in vivo). Horm Metab Res. 1987 Jun;19(6):233-8. doi: 10.1055/s-2007-1011788. PubMed PMID: 2887500.

[80] Chattopadhyay S, Raychaudhuri U, Chakraborty R. Artificial sweeteners – a review. J Food Sci Technol. 2014 Apr;51(4):611-21. doi: 10.1007/s13197-011-0571-1. Epub 2011 Oct 21. Review. PubMed PMID: 24741154; PubMed Central PMCID: PMC3982014.

[81] Pepino MY, Tiemann CD, Patterson BW, Wice BM, Klein S. Sucralose affects glycemic and hormonal responses to an oral glucose load. Diabetes Care. 2013 Sep;36(9):2530-5. doi: 10.2337/dc12-2221. Epub 2013 Apr 30. PubMed PMID: 23633524; PubMed Central PMCID: PMC3747933.

[82] Anton SD, Martin CK, Han H, Coulon S, Cefalu WT, Geiselman P, Williamson DA. Effects of stevia, aspartame, and sucrose on food intake, satiety, and postprandial glucose and insulin levels. Appetite. 2010 Aug;55(1):37-43. doi: 10.1016/j.appet.2010.03.009. Epub 2010 Mar 18. PubMed PMID: 20303371; PubMed Central PMCID: PMC2900484.

[83] Tey SL, Salleh NB, Henry J, Forde CG. Effects of aspartame-, monk fruit-, stevia- and sucrose-sweetened beverages on postprandial glucose, insulin and energy intake. Int J Obes (Lond). 2017 Mar;41(3):450-457. doi: 10.1038/ijo.2016.225. Epub 2016 Dec 13. PubMed PMID: 27956737.

[84] Jeppesen PB, Gregersen S, Poulsen CR, Hermansen K. Stevioside acts directly on pancreatic beta cells to secrete insulin: actions independent of cyclic adenosine monophosphate and adenosine triphosphate-sensitive K+-channel activity. Metabolism. 2000 Feb;49(2):208-14. doi: 10.1016/s0026-0495(00)91325-8. PubMed PMID: 10690946.

[85] Bhasker S, Madhav H, Chinnamma M. Molecular evidence of insulinomimetic property exhibited by steviol and stevioside in diabetes induced L6 and 3T3L1 cells. Phytomedicine. 2015 Oct 15;22(11):1037-44. doi: 10.1016/j.phymed.2015.07.007. Epub 2015 Aug 14. PubMed PMID: 26407946.

[86] Tey SL, Salleh NB, Henry J, Forde CG. Effects of aspartame-, monk fruit-, stevia- and sucrose-sweetened beverages on postprandial glucose, insulin and energy intake. Int J Obes (Lond). 2017 Mar;41(3):450-457. doi: 10.1038/ijo.2016.225. Epub 2016 Dec 13. PubMed PMID: 27956737.

[87] Zhou Y, Zheng Y, Ebersole J, Huang CF. Insulin secretion stimulating effects of mogroside V and fruit extract of luo han kuo (Siraitia grosvenori Swingle) fruit extract.. Yao Xue Xue Bao. 2009 Nov;44(11):1252-7. PubMed PMID: 21351724.

[88] Yang Q. Gain weight by "going diet?" Artificial sweeteners and the neurobiology of sugar cravings: Neuroscience 2010. Yale J Biol Med. 2010 Jun;83(2):101-8. PMID: 20589192; PMCID: PMC2892765.

[89] Anton SD, Martin CK, Han H, Coulon S, Cefalu WT, Geiselman P, Williamson DA. Effects of stevia, aspartame, and sucrose on food intake, satiety, and postprandial glucose and insulin levels. Appetite. 2010 Aug;55(1):37-43. doi: 10.1016/j.appet.2010.03.009. Epub 2010 Mar 18. PubMed PMID: 20303371; PubMed Central PMCID: PMC2900484.

[90] Liang Y, Steinbach G, Maier V, Pfeiffer EF. The effect of artificial sweetener on insulin secretion. 1. The effect of acesulfame K on insulin secretion in the rat (studies in vivo). Horm Metab Res. 1987 Jun;19(6):233-8. doi: 10.1055/s-2007-1011788. PubMed PMID: 2887500.

[91] Yang Q. Gain weight by "going diet?" Artificial sweeteners and the neurobiology of sugar cravings: Neuroscience 2010. Yale J Biol Med. 2010 Jun;83(2):101-8. PMID: 20589192; PMCID: PMC2892765.

[92] Bellisle F, Drewnowski A. Intense sweeteners, energy intake and the control of body weight. Eur J Clin Nutr. 2007 Jun;61(6):691-700. doi: 10.1038/sj.ejcn.1602649. Epub 2007 Feb 7. Review. PubMed PMID: 17299484.

[93] Ruiz-Ojeda FJ, Plaza-Díaz J, Sáez-Lara MJ, Gil A. Effects of Sweeteners on the Gut Microbiota: A Review of Experimental Studies and Clinical Trials. Adv Nutr. 2019 Jan 1;10(suppl_1):S31-S48. doi: 10.1093/advances/nmy037. PubMed PMID: 30721958; PubMed Central PMCID: PMC6363527.

[94] Abou-Donia MB, El-Masry EM, Abdel-Rahman AA, McLendon RE, Schiffman SS. Splenda alters gut microflora and increases intestinal p-glycoprotein and cytochrome p-450 in male rats. J Toxicol Environ Health A. 2008;71(21):1415-29. doi: 10.1080/15287390802328630. PubMed PMID: 18800291.

[95] Pepino MY, Tiemann CD, Patterson BW, Wice BM, Klein S. Sucralose affects glycemic and hormonal responses to an oral glucose load. Diabetes Care. 2013 Sep;36(9):2530-5. doi: 10.2337/dc12-2221. Epub 2013 Apr 30. PubMed PMID: 23633524; PubMed Central PMCID: PMC3747933.

[96] Nuttall FQ, Gannon MC. Plasma glucose and insulin response to macronutrients in nondiabetic and NIDDM subjects. Diabetes Care. 1991 Sep;14(9):824-38. doi: 10.2337/diacare.14.9.824. Review. PubMed PMID: 1959475.

[97] Li X, Chen H, Guan Y, Li X, Lei L, Liu J, Yin L, Liu G, Wang Z. Acetic acid activates the AMP-activated protein kinase signaling pathway to regulate lipid metabolism in bovine hepatocytes. PLoS One. 2013;8(7):e67880. doi: 10.1371/journal.pone.0067880. Print 2013. PubMed PMID: 23861826; PubMed Central PMCID: PMC3701595.

[98]Eat This Much Inc [Internet]. California: Redondo Beach; c2018 [cited 2021 Jan 29]. Available from: https://www.eatthismuch.com/food/nutrition/exogenous-ketones,2713557/.

[99]Corrao G, Rubbiati L, Bagnardi V, Zambon A, Poikolainen K. Alcohol and coronary heart disease: a meta-analysis. Addiction. 2000    Oct;95(10):1505-23. doi:                10.1046/j.1360-0443.2000.951015056.x. PubMed PMID: 11070527.

[100]Yuan JM, Ross RK, Gao YT, Henderson BE, Yu MC. Follow up study of moderate alcohol intake and mortality among middle aged men in Shanghai, China. BMJ. 1997    Jan    4;314(7073):18-23. doi: 10.1136/bmj.314.7073.18. PubMed        PMID: 9001474; PubMed Central PMCID: PMC2125578.

[101]Shai I, Wainstein J, Harman-Boehm I, Raz I, Fraser D, Rudich A, Stampfer MJ. Glycemic effects of moderate alcohol intake among patients with type 2 diabetes: a multicenter, randomized, clinical intervention trial. Diabetes Care. 2007  Dec;30(12):3011-6. doi: 10.2337/dc07-1103. Epub 2007 Sep 11. PubMed PMID: 17848609.

[102]Napoli R, Cozzolino D, Guardasole V, Angelini V, Zarra E, Matarazzo M, Cittadini A, Saccà L, Torella R. Red wine consumption improves insulin resistance but not endothelial function in type 2 diabetic patients. Metabolism. 2005 Mar;54(3):306-13. doi:      10.1016/j.metabol.2004.09.010.      PMID: 15736107.

[103] Park D, Jeong H, Lee MN, Koh A, Kwon O, Yang YR, Noh J, Suh PG, Park H, Ryu SH. Resveratrol induces autophagy by directly inhibiting mTOR through ATP competition. Sci Rep. 2016 Feb 23;6:21772. doi: 10.1038/srep21772. PubMed PMID: 26902888; PubMed Central PMCID: PMC4763238.

[104] White AM, Johnston CS. Vinegar ingestion at bedtime moderates waking glucose concentrations in adults with well-controlled type 2 diabetes. Diabetes Care. 2007 Nov;30(11):2814-5. doi: 10.2337/dc07-1062. Epub 2007 Aug 21. PubMed PMID: 17712024.

[105] Petsiou EI, Mitrou PI, Raptis SA, Dimitriadis GD. Effect and mechanisms of action of vinegar on glucose metabolism, lipid profile, and body weight. Nutr Rev. 2014 Oct;72(10):651-61. doi: 10.1111/nure.12125. Epub 2014 Aug 28. Review. PubMed PMID: 25168916.

[106] Li X, Chen H, Guan Y, Li X, Lei L, Liu J, Yin L, Liu G, Wang Z. Acetic acid activates the AMP-activated protein kinase signaling pathway to regulate lipid metabolism in bovine hepatocytes. PLoS One. 2013;8(7):e67880. doi: 10.1371/journal.pone.0067880. Print 2013. PubMed PMID: 23861826; PubMed Central PMCID: PMC3701595.

[107] Petsiou EI, Mitrou PI, Raptis SA, Dimitriadis GD. Effect and mechanisms of action of vinegar on glucose metabolism, lipid profile, and body weight. Nutr Rev. 2014 Oct;72(10):651-61. doi: 10.1111/nure.12125. Epub 2014 Aug 28. Review. PubMed PMID: 25168916.

[108] *The Self NutritionData method and system [Internet]. New York: Condé Nast; c2018 [cited 2021 Jan 29]. Available from: https://nutritiondata.self.com/facts/beverages/3965/2.*

[109] *Prasanth MI, Sivamaruthi BS, Chaiyasut C, Tencomnao T. A Review of the Role of Green Tea (Camellia sinensis) in Antiphotoaging, Stress Resistance, Neuroprotection, and Autophagy. Nutrients. 2019 Feb 23;11(2). doi: 10.3390/nu11020474. Review. PubMed PMID: 30813433; PubMed Central PMCID: PMC6412948.*

# About the Author

Never before had people paid more attention to their diet and prioritized exercise than today. Nevertheless, diseases caused by diet and lifestyle are increasing from year to year.

Since the food and pharmaceutical industries still predominantly influence dietary guidelines and tell us what is healthy, Stephan Lederer made it his mission to counteract these contradictions.

On www.mentalfoodchain.com, he curates one of the fastest-growing independent health blogs.

In doing so, Stephan is the first blogger and author who, as part of his data-driven approach, rejects mere assertions and instead always shows the current state of research based on studies.

His online archive offers concentrated knowledge about intermittent fasting, the keto diet, and the hormones behind it, which control our everyday life based on diet and lifestyle.

The author's stated goal is to equip readers with the knowledge that will get them in the physical and mental shape their loved ones deserve, without having to count calories or exercise daily.

# What Can You Drink During Intermittent Fasting?

What Can You Drink During Intermittent Fasting?

## Disclaimer

The contents of this book have been checked and pre-pared with great care. However, the author cannot guar-antee or warranty the contents' completeness, accuracy, and timeliness.

The content of this book represents the personal experi-ence and opinion of the author and is intended for infor-mational and entertainment purposes only. Therefore, no legal responsibility or guarantee for the success of the mentioned tips and advice can be assumed. The author assumes no responsibility for the non-achievement of the goals described in the book.

This book contains links to other websites. The author has no influence on the content of these websites. Therefore, the author cannot take responsibility for this content. The respective provider or operator of the pages is responsible for the content of the linked pages. Illegal contents could not be determined at the time of linking.

What Can You Drink During Intermittent Fasting?

What Can You Drink During Intermittent Fasting?

## Contact

What Can You Drink During Intermittent Fasting?

The Science of Fasting Explained

1. Edition

ISBN: 9798473191769

Mag. Stephan Lederer, Bakk., MSc, Sigmundstadl 20/3, AT-8020 Graz

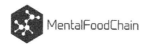

www.mentalfoodchain.com

Printed in Great Britain
by Amazon

67015038R00078